WISDOM FROM THE WOMB

The Magic of a Baby-Led Birth

GENEVA MONTANO, CPM

www.genevamontano.com

Birth photography credits:

      Aperture Grrl Photography
      Rebecca Ann Walsh Photography/Birth Becomes Her
      Taylor Davenport Photography
      Forest Joy, Moon Child Doula

Disclaimer: This is a work of nonfiction. The people and events described are real, and I have permission to use my version of their stories. I recognize that their versions might be different than my own. Although I am a Certified Professional Midwife and a Certified Doula, I am not your care provider. I am not providing advice, medical or otherwise, simply presenting information. This information cannot replace the advice of a competent care provider and your own intuition.

PRINT ISBN 979-8-6400-5855-0

This book is dedicated to my greatest teachers, the four infinite beings who chose me to be their mother, and to Ella Blu

CONTENTS

Foreword 7

Midwife Life.. 15

    Womb Connection: Journey to your Baby........................... 32

Wisdom from the Womb.. 34

    Womb Connection: Practice Listening 50

    Womb Wisdom: Caroline's Story 52

Finding My Own Womb Wisdom 56

    Womb Connection: What Did your Birth Stories Teach You?
....73

Seeing Cycles 74

    Womb Connection: Noticing Cycles...................................76

    Fear-Tension-Pain Cycle 77

    Womb Connection: What Does your Baby Need Now?....... 84

    Womb Connection: Breath of Light 94

    Cosmic Breath 3... 95

    Womb Wisdom: Dace's Story.. 96

Facing Fear 101

    Womb Connection: Fear Balancing Kriya...........................129

    Womb Connection: Following your Fears 130

    Womb Wisdom: Jakota's Story 131

The Preparations: What Really Matters 135

    Womb Connection: Channeling the Mother Goddess 152

Preparing Your Body for Birth.......................................154

    Womb Connection: Kriyas 164

    Physical Fitness 166

Womb Connection: Pelvic Bowl Sweep 176

Womb Connection: Perineal Massage 178

Preparing Your Mind, Heart, and Spirit for Birth.................... 181

Womb Connection: Ho'oponopono 188

Womb Connection: Journey to your Fetal Self 190

Womb Wisdom: Jaclyn's Story 192

The Passage 196

Womb Connection: Exploring Your Anatomy.................. 203

Womb Connection: Giving Gratitude to your Organs 204

Womb Connection: Shifting Adrenaline to Oxytocin.......... 211

Womb Connection: Early Labor: Letter to your Baby 228

Womb Connection: Find a Mantra 232

Womb Connection: Finding your Voice Intimacy Play 243

Womb Connection: Lion's Breath...................................... 244

Womb Connection—Rolling the Dice 245

Womb Wisdom: Marion's Story 247

The Decisions: (aka Informed Choice) 252

Womb Connection.. 294

Cascade of Interventions Card Game 294

Womb Wisdom: Alex's Story 297

The Return (aka Your Postpartum Time)............................. 302

Womb Connection: Pelvic-Floor Breathing....................... 317

The Magic of a Baby-Led Birth 318

Acknowledgments... 328

About the Author 329

Resources Mentioned 331

Endnotes 332

FOREWORD

WHEN GENEVA ASKED ME to write the foreword to her book, saying that I felt honored is an understatement. I don't just say this as her writing coach or as an author myself. I say this, first and foremost, as a former client who experienced firsthand the magic Geneva embodies in her approach to birth.

My pregnancy was... a surprise. I had never been one of those people who dreamed of each and every detail up to the moment I had a child. At a certain point, I wasn't even sure if I would or could have a child.

When I found out I was carrying a life inside me, I did the only thing I knew how to do up to that point: *plan*. Just like I had made a plan for every detail in my professional life, I would do the same for my baby. Part of that plan was finding a doula to help me through the details of this plan. I wanted a home birth and my partner wanted a hospital birth, so we compromised with a gentle hospital delivery following the hypnobirthing protocol, avoiding drugs and medical intervention at all costs. I had interviewed two doulas before Geneva. When she and I met at the third meeting, I knew she was the one who would usher my firstborn into the world, because she was also a very experienced midwife acting as a doula in my case to help me out. In addition to her certifications and decades of experience, there was just something about her that led me immediately to trust her.

I didn't know much about birth before the Universe brought Geneva into my life, but I sure thought I did (she is somewhere reading this, vigorously nodding her head in agreement); because everything we need to know about birth is found on the Internet, right? Wrong. So, so wrong.

Yes, we can find endless amounts of information through the Google machine, but what we don't find is any information on how to incorporate into our birthing experience the innate wisdom that already lives inside of all of us. And don't get me started on how the media portrays childbirth, with the screaming and sweating and wailing and terror of it all.

This is where Geneva's guidance began to shift my perspective on how my child would enter the world and open my mind to the possibility of a different experience than the ones I had seen on TV, one where I felt empowered and safe, creating my reality, instead of becoming a pawn in someone else's cookie-cutter protocol. Not to mention all of the knowledge Geneva introduced me to around the history of birth that grew my trust in myself and my child above all outside parties.

While I initially clung tight to my plan, my prenatal sessions with Geneva helped me gradually to let go of control over the being who had ultimate control over this birth: my son. She assisted me in releasing every story I'd ever heard about how birth was "supposed" to go, based on society and Obstetrics' depiction of the experience. Through her expertise, vast knowledge, gentle guidance, and her own innate intuitive wisdom, I eventually arrived at a place where I began to tune into my baby and trust that the plan he had was best for us both.

Spoiler alert: Things inevitably did *not* go according to [my original] plan. Funny how that works, huh? I remember my first call to Geneva after I went into labor, amidst my deep breaths and affirmations, and her sounding so calm, so peaceful, so still, so trusting on the other end. When I rolled into the hospital with a Tupperware trunk full of household items to replicate my "homebirth," she didn't say one word, just smirked at me. It's like she knew exactly what I was about to discover through this experience.

I'm sure she thought to herself, "Oh, the founder of *The Less Effect* sure comes with a lot of baggage... literally!" I laugh at this now, as someone who prides herself in detachment from all things, not to mention transitioning from relying on the outside world to trusting wholeheartedly that we have everything we need inside of us. But, of course, the Universe always helps us out by really bringing home these messages we need to hear. And boy, was this reaffirmation clear when everything decided to take a different route.

While Geneva had imparted on me more than enough information and guidance on preparation for my body, fetal positioning, finding care providers, and all of my options at the hospital, when it came time for my son to make his appearance, she embodied ultimate surrender. It immediately put me at ease, and I followed suit, which, if you know anything about birth, you know is *extremely* important in opening up the birth passageway.

In the moments I would stray, she gently guided me back to myself and my body, encouraging me to be the observer of this miracle that was unfolding before me. Those were the moments I felt the most safe and the most in trust—and this is what my experience became. As experienced and knowledgeable as Geneva is, she approached my birth with a quiet confidence of knowing that, no matter how much information she or I had, ultimately, it was my baby who was in charge and her only job was to keep me in remembrance of this.

I don't believe my birth story would be complete without noting that, although I had progressed to ten centimeters beautifully and naturally without drugs or complications and my body began pushing on its own, just like Geneva taught me it would, it decided to keep pushing for 12 hours. Yes—I was in second-stage labor and pushing for 12 hours. I know now that this is unheard of. But, at the time, even though it was hard, my body just kept doing it! My sweet son's head was even showing. I know this because everyone in the room kept telling me how close he was... for 12 hours.

I recall, at hour 10 and still no drugs (God help me), the new obstetrician on duty came in and expressed concern for my baby's oxygen levels and offered an epidural to relax and hopefully allow this little human to come on out, despite my fervent request not to speak the "E" word.

This is the moment I knew I needed to go deeper into surrender and let go; not because I didn't have a choice, but because my baby was desperately trying to come out, and what we were doing wasn't working. I wouldn't have been surprised if we'd seen a hand pop out, waving at us as a gesture to get the Earth party started! I remember them administering the epidural and my taking the biggest sigh of relief of my life as I melted into the bed.

Once I was able to catch my breath, I scanned the room to see if I could spot Geneva amongst the sea of doctors and nurses, to thank her for spending so much time with me (plus all the work I was putting her through, all 135 naked pounds of me hanging all over her and primal moaning into her ear every 60 seconds for hours on end). I'll never forget finding her and noticing she was preparing to tuck me in, after everyone else left, to tell me to take a nap, then to tuck herself in a chair next to me, reassuring me that she wasn't going anywhere.

Shortly after, we started pushing again, and after 2 more hours, the doctor said we either needed to do a forceps delivery or a cesarean. I remember looking at Geneva for advice:

"Should I keep going? Should I stop? Should I take more drugs? Should I have them pry him out? Should I get cut open and just throw my entire birth plan out the window?"

While the choice to make was mine, thankfully, with Geneva's help, I had carved out an experience at a hospital that allowed for that choice. I reconnected with my baby like she had helped me do through my pregnancy.

What I heard was that he wanted to get out, but he needed help. So, I continued to put my ego and my precious birth plan aside and let them roll me into the operating room.

At that moment, I felt no fear of the unknown and zero shame about the deviation we were about to make, because I stayed in my power, using my baby as my north star through the entire experience—even if it wasn't what I had written down on a piece of paper for the entire hospital staff. The wisdom that Geneva helped me to uncover within my womb allowed me to remain calm and present among the uncertainty and to release the control, which allowed me to birth a healthy baby boy in the way it was always meant to happen.

When I read Geneva's final draft of her book, it brought me to tears. As an avid researcher/planner, I had read countless birthing books during my pregnancy, none of which taught me that I had any idea what I was doing. Instead, they overloaded me with voluminous data that I would not and could not remember, especially in the midst of what might be the most intense event of my life. It did the opposite of what I'm guessing they intended, by making me feel more out of touch with my body and my ability to do this thing called birth by exposing every bit of information I lacked.

In contrast, Geneva's powerful words, birth stories, clinical designations, and intuitive wisdom from the ancestors shines a bright light on the original birthplace of birth, a time when birthing people trusted their bodies, their babies, and their intrinsic ability to become one through the entire experience.

To any birthing person reading this book: be prepared for your view of birth to be forever changed. While you will receive important prenatal and childbirth information to allow you to prepare, it is delivered in a way that is tied to your inner-knowing, paired with methods to amplify that inner voice. As you dive deeper and deeper into this text, you will feel closer and closer to the being growing inside of you, and your confidence will grow right alongside them. It is a body of work that leaves birthing people with the greatest sense of wisdom they have ever known, empowered to the point of no return.

Wisdom from the Womb is a powerfully healing, full-circle moment for me—to have had Geneva's intuitive heart and healing hands guide my son through his own birth, and now, in return, to hold a similar space for her soul-work through the birth of this masterpiece. It brings me back to the place of knowing that all of the answers I ever needed were found right inside me the entire time, right inside my womb.

Samantha Joy
#1 Bestselling Author, *The Less Effect: Design Your Life for Happiness and Purpose*
International Identity Coach
Proud Mother to Landon Hail

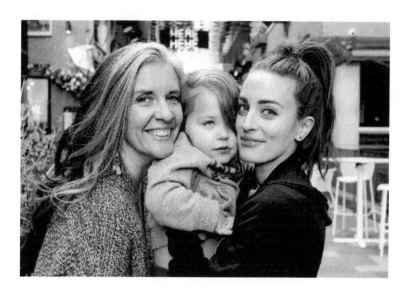

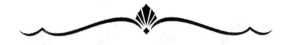

MIDWIFE LIFE

IT IS DECEMBER 29. It is quiet and dark, bitter cold outside in Denver, Colorado.

I'm snuggled under my covers, wishing for sleep. Every now and again, I hear my daughters playing downstairs, and I think I should probably go tell them it's time for bed, but my body is heavy. I have supported three births since Christmas day.

Today, I visited a sweet baby who was born at 12:02 a.m. on the 26th and his warrior mama in the NICU at Children's Hospital. He is so perfect, with curly black hair and the most beautiful caramel skin, and his little feet have the tiniest little jelly-bean toes that remind me of a tiny tiger. He doesn't cry much, but when he does, I feel the power in it. I feel him saying he is strong and he has something to teach us.

Brasahn is Emem's third baby. Her first was born by cesarean after a so-called "failed induction." Her second was a VBAC (Vaginal Birth After Cesarean) in the hospital, and she has always believed her babies should be born at home. Her family comes from Nigeria and for generations were supported by midwives to have their babies at home, surrounded by family. Emem's hope for this birth was to be supported by her husband and for him to catch the baby with my guidance. Her mother and sister would be downstairs watching her older two children, so they could all join us once the baby was born.

Emem's pregnancy was not the smoothest or easiest. In the beginning of the third trimester, her blood pressure started rising. We had hard conversations about her life, the stresses of being a black woman in America, her diet, sleep, exercise, and her heart's desire to have this baby at home. Her baby was not easy to palpate, even as he grew bigger, which made it difficult for a high-touch, low-tech care provider like myself to determine the position of a baby. I suspect he was breech until late in her pregnancy.

She cried on more than one occasion in my office when she thought about the prospect of having to go to the hospital to birth this baby. She felt a deep connection with her baby and she knew in her bones that her baby wanted to be born at home, just as much as she wanted him to be.

When he was breech, I suggested that she talk to her baby, visualize him head down, and clear up anything in her life that had a feeling of being upside down. She did just that. She talked to her baby, and the next time I saw her, the baby was head down.

Later in pregnancy, I could not determine by palpation or auscultation of heart tones whether or not he had remained head down, so she told him he needed to let me feel him and know where he was, and from that visit forward, even though Emem's own bodily tissue had grown larger—she was a plus size woman even before her pregnancies—I could always feel exactly where baby was.

As her blood pressure rose, she told her baby he needed to help her be healthy and she says she made a deal with him that she would not have preeclampsia. I drew labs to rule out this high-risk disorder of pregnancy, and her blood did not show the telltale signs of preeclampsia. But it did show she was slightly anemic and that her body could use more nourishment at two weeks before her due date.

We created a diet plan with high-protein foods, nourishing leafy greens, and teas, and no processed foods whatsoever. I told her we would redraw the labs in one week, and if they were not within normal limits, she would be considered high risk and we would transfer care to an OB. I was uncertain if one week would be enough time to change the levels we were seeing in her blood. Emem did not seem discouraged at all though. She put her hand on her full, round belly and spoke to her son, telling him he needed to wait until her body was well-nourished and balanced for birth. Her hopes manifested in her body. Emem's labs came back normal at the next blood draw. Her blood pressure never got too high. Her wish for a home birth was still possible.

Her due date came and went, and while my midwife heart struggled not to get caught in anxious places, Emem never seemed worried at all. She told me she kept seeing the number 26, and so she was pretty sure he would come that day. Despite anything that came up, she never stopped trusting that her baby wanted to be born at home.

I did not have big plans on Christmas, and if I have a day with not much to do, the universe will usually fill that time for me with a birth. I texted her that morning, nothing about labor, but I was hoping if I checked in, she might let me know if she was rumbling at all. Her response just told me to have a wonderful Christmas, but nothing of having contractions. So I went on about my day, and so did she.

Little did I know, she was having irregular contractions all day, and after 9 p.m., she went for a walk to try to increase the contractions and tell her baby it was time to come. She told him to come right into his dad's hands on the 26th. Her labor picked up but she waited a little while to call me, to make sure labor was well established. When her husband called to say she was in labor, I could hear Emem's birth song in the background and I jumped out of bed, pulled on my scrubs, packed up the car and started driving to her house, whispering a prayer for this birth.

Brasahn was born seven minutes later! Right into his dad's hands at 12:02am on the 26th. I was in my car but nowhere close to their house when I received their second call saying that baby had been born.

Emem and her husband were both joyous and joking, thrilled to meet their sweet baby, who was doing perfectly, and in shock that things had happened so quickly. I stayed on the phone with them until I arrived at their house. A while later, the placenta was born. I cleaned up, and checked baby and mom head to toe. They were both healthy and happy, with perfect vital signs. Baby was covered in vernix and lanugo. He had cupid's bow lips and clear, wise, dark eyes. He looked around at this world with curiosity and appeared to love feeling safe snuggled next to his mom, skin to skin. He nursed right away and cried when anyone disturbed his happy suckling. His grandma and auntie came, and the love and joy that surrounded this amazing birth was palpable.

We stayed for several hours after the birth, and then returned the next day for a routine follow-up visit. I performed Brasahn's routine newborn screenings, the Newborn Metabolic Screen, and the CCHD screening, which screens for a congenital heart defect. Brasahn's numbers were not quite where they needed to be on the CCHD screening. A repeat test an hour later confirmed this.

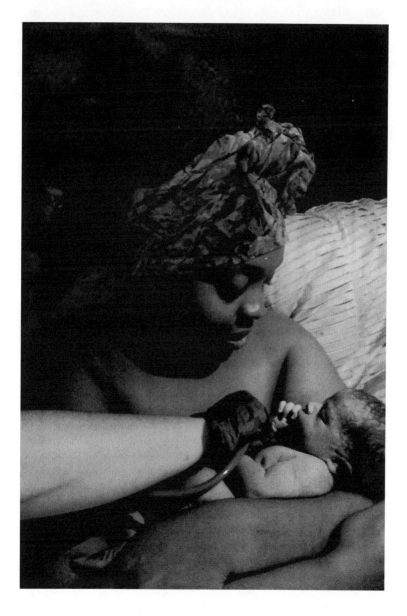

It felt perplexing, because he seemed so perfect. He was nursing well, he was pink and alert, his heart and lungs sounded normal—he looked like every other normal healthy baby I have taken care of.

I recommended they get ahold of their pediatrician, but it was a Friday afternoon, and the doctors were out of the office. I called a few friendly docs I know in the area, and they both recommended that Emem take the baby to the ER. She wasn't very happy about this idea and was leaning toward waiting until she could go see her own pediatrician Monday morning, standing in full faith that her sweet boy was perfect. Everything felt confusing and chaotic to the family and to me. After praying, connecting with her baby, and some tough conversations, Emem decided to take her baby to the ER. We all expected that the doctors would say the baby is fine, go home. But the next call I received was Emem saying they were transporting her perfect baby to Children's Hospital by ambulance for specialized testing. I felt shocked, humbled, and worried, while hoping for the best as I lay my head down to rest after this whirlwind of a day.

A few hours later, I got a call that Stephanie was in labor. Stephanie had planned her first birth at a freestanding birth center. During her first labor, her water broke at home at almost 42 weeks, and she had a very long, hard labor during which she was sent home a few times and eventually sent to the hospital for failure to progress. Her baby was occiput posterior, which is a non-optimal position for the baby and generally causes a longer labor with more frequent and more painful contractions. At the hospital she got an epidural, Pitocin, pushed for several hours, and eventually gave birth by cesarean two days after she had gone into labor. Stephanie is such a strong woman. After experiencing a birth like this, I know she can do anything she puts her mind to.

With her second baby, hoping for a very different experience—she planned a home vaginal birth after cesarean (HBAC). She paid close attention to her body mechanics and got chiropractic treatment throughout pregnancy. She was very connected to her baby—always aware of where her baby was in her body. At the end of her third trimester, Stephanie was struggling with keeping up with her self-care and reducing stress. She got a message from her baby that she should work less and take Christmas week off. What do you know, she went into labor at 39 weeks.

I made my way over to Stephanie's house where I found her having strong contractions every three minutes on her hands and knees, her TENS unit sending gentle electrical impulses into her lower back muscles. Her husband was really nervous about home birth. His mother is a doctor, and he believes strongly in Western medicine. After seeing his first child's birth, when he also didn't get to sleep for two days, he was skeptical that having a baby at home would be a good plan.

Stephanie was the picture of grace and confidence. She knew this birth was going to be different. From the moment I met her, she never doubted her body or her baby. Though I have to imagine somewhere within her she knew there was a possibility that things could end in a repeat cesarean, I believe she would have handled that with an equal amount of grace and confidence. But that was not her story. At her house, I suggested she try standing or sitting on the toilet for a little while, but she was not excited about moving. Hands and knees was what felt good to her and where her baby wanted to be. So she stayed on her hands and knees.

Eventually, I did convince her that maybe walking to the toilet to empty her bladder might be a good idea. When she got there, she decided she would try sitting there for a few more contractions, and she ended up really liking the toilet. I was in the bathroom with her, listening to heart tones, and noticing that her body was pushing spontaneously with contractions, when her water broke on the toilet.

Her water had meconium in it. After the next contraction, I started to tell her the risks and protocols associated with meconium, but just then she roared the roar that every midwife knows brings a baby. I asked her to touch inside her vagina, and she felt her baby's head just inside. She was certain she did not want to walk to the living room to get into birth pool, which we had just finished filling for the water birth she had planned. Instead, she took one step in front of the toilet and got back on her hands and knees. Her baby's favorite position.

Her husband Peter and I were in the tiny bathroom with her and the back end of her body. My assistants and her sister were in the hallway with her head and the front end of her body. And in four more pushes, she had an amazing baby girl.

Peter caught her and handed her through to Stephanie, who seemed not one bit surprised she had just had a VBAC at home. She knew she would do it. She trusted her baby and her body and knew with her whole being that this baby would be born at home, naturally.

I was ecstatic for her. Thrilled that she got to experience a peaceful home birth after the disappointment she had expressed with her first. I think I was more excited than she was. Her demeanor was nothing other than, "I knew I could do this." What a badass. We cleaned up and checked everyone out. It was about 7:30 a.m. and snowing hard when my team and I left Stephanie's house.

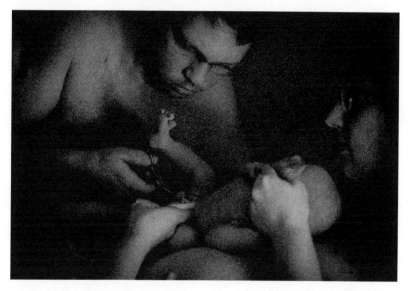

I went home and slept for a few hours then got up and cleaned my house, which was still in a post-holiday state of craze. I saw a client at my home office who was officially 39 weeks that day, and then went to teach an Infant CPR class.

After class, I came home and passed out for about an hour but had trouble sleeping, which made no sense, since I had not slept much the last few nights. I was restless. I knew that a family I was acting as doula for was in the hospital being induced, and my doula partner was planning to attend her birth. There were lots of texts back and forth on a group thread about how things were going, and the birthing person said she thought she would not need anyone until morning.

I finally dozed off around 2:30 a.m. but was awakened

by a phone call from my partner asking if I could go support the laboring family for four or five hours. She would take over later in the morning. I somehow dragged myself out of bed and headed to the hospital to support Cammie.

Cammie is forty-two years old. This would be her first birth after fifteen pregnancies that all ended in loss. My mind cannot even wrap itself around these numbers. I feel an ache in my heart just telling her truth. I am in awe of how strong she is. How strong women are. That we don't just give up and die from the pain that is carried in our bodies from the losses we experience. That we can lose a child or experience disrespect and trauma in the most vulnerable moments of our lives, and somehow, we keep going. I am in awe that she trusts this baby will be born healthy. It would be so tempting just to be afraid.

Cammie does not really care how her baby gets here, as long as he gets here. She felt strongly that her baby would be safest if she was induced at 37 weeks. It is usually recommended to wait until 39 weeks for the best outcomes. Cammie's baby told her he was ready now. After laboring beautifully for several hours unmedicated through the early hours of the morning, Cammie was ready to get an epidural. After she was comfortable and ready to get some sleep, the nurse checked her and she was still 1-2 cm. Getting an epidural was the perfect choice for her and her baby. They decided to start Pitocin, and Cammie recommended I go home. She felt comfortable being at the hospital, just her and her husband, now that she was comfortable. She would call my doula partner later, when she needed more assistance. She is still in labor as I type this. She is feeling good, excited to meet her baby, who is handling labor well, and the texts back and forth on the group thread continue.

I left the hospital, went to check on Stephanie and her baby, who were doing wonderfully. Peter said to me as we were carrying the birth pool out to my car, "Thanks for making a believer out of me."

Oh, those are the moments that make my midwife heart melt. *Thank you*, Peter, for being willing to support your warrior wife in having the birth she knew she could have, even though it was uncomfortable for you. I am humbled by your trust in your wife and your baby, when you didn't truly trust birth, and you were pretty skeptical of me, as well. I am happy that the first thing your baby felt when she was born was your hands, even when I noticed you glance at your hands in disbelief, and a little bit of concern at the blood covering them.

Next stop, Children's Hospital. I know Emem hasn't slept much. Her mom is at the hospital with her, and her husband is struggling. He does not agree with the care the doctors are recommending, so rather than argue, he left to go be with the other boys at home. She hasn't eaten yet today, but she doesn't want me to pick anything up, as she says she will get something from the cafeteria.

I arrive to a dark room. Emem is sitting up, holding Brasahn in her arms. He is swaddled and has a CPAP mask taped to his face and a tube taped into his mouth. I can't see them, but she says there is an IV in his arm and one in his umbilical cord. He is still the cutest, sweetest little angel.

I sit with them, talk to them. She tells me that they have given her a diagnosis, but that she is rebuking this diagnosis. She believes her baby will be a medical miracle, and when they repeat his testing tomorrow, they will be shocked to learn that his diagnosis is incorrect and he is strong and ready to go home. This is her Truth in this moment.

I gave her some Arnica and Rescue Remedy to calm her nervous system and talked to her about taking care of herself, eating and drinking and resting. I can see she cannot rest because her spirit is fighting so hard for her son. When I say this to her, she starts to cry but quickly fights back her tears and says, since Brasahn isn't crying, she won't either.

I heard once that they found the same cancer-curing substances that are in breast milk in a mother's tears, and I share with Emem that her tears can help heal her child's heart and her heart. She looks so beautiful, holding her baby and sitting squarely in trust that her baby is perfect.

I say a prayer for Brasahn, silently, with one hand on his heart and one on hers. I have a vision of miniature angels dropping a shiny, new, red, glowing heart into his chest. She tells him over and over again how strong he is and how she knows he is meant for great things on this earth. Things like playing with his brothers, laughing, letting things be easy.

She tells him she trusts him. That throughout her pregnancy, she always trusted him. She always knew he would listen to her. When she needed him head down, he turned. When she needed him to wait, he waited. When she told him to come straight into his dad's hands, he did it right away. She wanted a home birth so much, and she is so happy she had one, saying that no one can ever take that magical experience from them. She trusted her baby would be born in the perfect way, and she believes with her entire being that he was. She trusts him even now, that he is okay, and that he is healthy and strong.

I cry healing mama tears for her. Again, humbled at the strength and trust that women possess. They know what is true for them and their babies, against all odds.

***

Who am I to be offered the gift of supporting these warrior women through these experiences? Who am I to witness the strength and grace it takes for a woman to face her fears, face death, and be reborn through the birth of her child? Who am I?

First and foremost, I am a divine creation of God, as is every being on this planet. Secondly, I am a divine creator, as is every being on this planet. However, in addition to my birthright as a creator, I also happen to be a mother. I have cradled life in my womb seven times. I have four amazing children, who are my biggest teachers and my biggest blessings in this life.

Third, I am a midwife. I have always been a midwife in this lifetime, and I believe have been a midwife in many lifetimes. In the time and place I live, people think of a midwife as a care provider who has gone through nursing school and done additional schooling, to have the certification to catch babies in the hospital or a birth center. Many people don't know what a midwife is at all.

My heart says that midwives are so much more than just someone who checks your blood pressure and catches your baby. I think back to villages where the survival of a people depended on their reproduction and on healthy moms and healthy babies. I think about how their health was so much more than physical, in that time. They believed the divine controlled their lives and their paths. They believed plants held medicine and could work on their behalf. They believed women's bodies were sacred and magical and powerful and that babies hold wisdom, as well. That their births told the story of their pasts and their futures.

The midwives were the keepers of the secrets surrounding birth, and therefore life. They held the mystery and the magic of portals opening as new souls made their way into this dimension, and sometimes out, too. Midwives were honored medicine women, priestesses, and gatekeepers. They were the grandmothers, the caretakers of families, and they were the witches who were burned at the stake. They were the women who hid their wisdom, quietly passing it down to the next generation, so as not to have it lost forever. In my heart, that is who I am. Beyond checking blood pressure and catching babies, I see birth as so much more than a means to get the baby out. I see the birthing people as divine vessels of creation. In every birth and every birthing person and every baby, I see miracles.

I started doing birth work in 2004, after the birth of my second child. I have since attended over 650 births. I have had a deep connection with God and the divine, and a desire to help people heal the wounds of their hearts and spirits my entire life.

I practice and teach yoga, not just as a physical practice, but as a way to create union between the body, mind, spirit, and the divine. I offer healing sessions to the people I serve that combine body work, energy work, plant medicine, chakra balancing, belief clearing, and whatever else I am guided to do. Besides being a born healer, I have trained under many pastors, gurus, energy workers, shamanic practitioners, herbalists, and priestesses.

I do not claim to have any answers or knowledge that has not already been provided in some other form about birth. The thing is, birth doesn't change! The protocols and technology supporting birth are constantly changing, but the wise woman's knowledge of birth has always and will always remain the same. I do not claim to have some newfangled way to keep you from feeling pain during your birth or save you from surgery. In fact, I believe that pain is part of the process and sometimes surgery is part of your baby's unique journey into this world. Nothing I state in this book should be taken as medical advice. No matter what anyone tells you, checking with your intuition and a trusted care provider before making a decision about your birth or your baby is wise. This book is simply a collection of some of the wisdom and stories I have collected over the years. My hope is that, in reading it, you will gain some glimmer of the magic and the wisdom that is held within you, that IS you! And that you can find more trust in birth, in yourself, in your baby, in the still small voices that guide you in your life and in your birth.

The truth is, there is no right way to have a baby. The bodies of biological female mammals are designed to give birth. It's literally written in our DNA to give birth. Where it gets tricky for humans is that we have free will. We have thoughts and emotions. History, trauma, and baggage. We have heard stories from our mothers and our friends and random women at the grocery store. We have seen terrible renditions of birth on TV. Human females have been programmed to distrust their bodies and their wisdom ever since the time they exited the womb themselves. So birth is not as straightforward as it may seem.

Our current culture relies heavily on knowledge and scientific data, over intuition and trust. Both are important when it comes to birth. But you can never have enough knowledge or facts to predict your birth. Learn all you can about birth; it is good to be prepared. Yet at the end of the day, what might matter most is to know it will be a unique journey between you and your unborn baby and all you really have to do is experience this journey. Truly be present and feel the excitement, the anticipation, the worry, and the joy. Truly connect and feel your baby. Birth is a wild ride.

Imagine what the world might be like if, no matter what that ride looked like, at every birth, a baby is surrounded by peace and love and is given the time it needs to transition to life Earth-side and is respected as an individual—even in utero; if every birthing person is given options and care that make them feel safe and special; and if every partner can see the raw power and beauty that comes out of the birthing person, as they roar their baby out. I believe women are creators and if they were cared for in the way they were meant to be, the world would change one birth, one baby, one family, one community at a time.

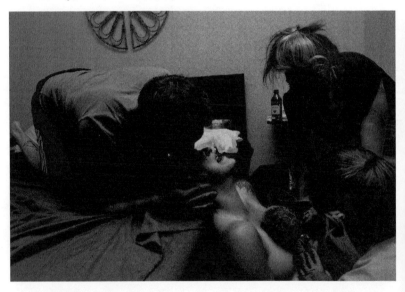

Unfortunately, no matter how much we believe this is true, in our current world this is not going to be every person's story. Birth is not always peaceful nor are women and babies always cared for in a way that leaves them feeling special and powerful. I find there is an epidemic of people who judge themselves harshly for the way their baby is born, blaming themselves somehow that things were not different. Sometimes, things happen that we cannot explain and no one can fix, despite everyone's best efforts.

Again, you cannot ever actually know enough or do enough preparation to control your birth experience. Birth is just like life. It will teach us what we need to learn, and we can go with the flow and accept it, or we can fight it along the way. We might be able to affect some of the turns it takes, but we can never control it.

We take the twists and turns of life assured of one outcome—death. We do our best to enjoy the journey and make decisions that will bring us the most love, peace, and contentment along the way, but we cannot actually plan or control how one single day will play out.

In birth, similarly, we are assured of one outcome—the baby will come out. The twists and turns are unknown. Try as we might to plan and control this time, birth (like life) has a known end, and everything else is an unknown variable. We can, however, enjoy the journey and make decisions that will bring us the most love, peace, and contentment along the way. We can create a loving and peaceful environment no matter how the baby comes out.

I wonder: how might this small shift change the world we live in?

***

A note about Womb Connections:
Each womb connection can be found on my website,
www.GenevaMontano.com/WisdomFromTheWomb
where I demonstrate the action, provide more
guidance, or talk you through a meditative journey.

***

WOMB CONNECTION
JOURNEY TO YOUR BABY

* Find a quiet place where you can lie down or sit down.

* Close your eyes, relax, and place one hand on your heart and one hand on your baby.

* Feel your breath. Each time you inhale, see your breath moving in through your nose, down your airway, into your lungs, and landing in your heart.

* See the energy of your heart as a small bright light, and see that light begin to grow. Notice what this light looks like. What color is your heart's light? How big does it want to become? Are there any spots on it that do not glow as bright?

* After you feel connected to your heart's light, begin to bring your breath into your womb. See the light of your baby's heart. Is it the same color as yours or different?

* See the light from your heart traveling down into your womb and connecting with your baby's heart.

* Now, start to see, feel, or imagine your heart's light swirling together with the light of your baby's heart. See how they combine and dance with one another. With each breath you take, feel the connection of your heart to your baby's heart.

* Feel your heartbeat under one hand and your belly rising and falling under your other hand and, with each breath, *Just BE...* Be with this amazing connection that is.

  With each breath, your heart is pumping blood and energy and light and love through your body, into your uterus, through the placenta into the baby's umbilical cord, all around baby's heart and body, back through the umbilical cord, the placenta, your uterus, and back to your heart. Every breath you take brings life to your baby.

* When you feel complete and connected to your baby, give gratitude to your baby and tuck their light back into their heart.

* Then, see your own light tuck back into your own heart. Give your heart gratitude for all the work it does every minute.

* Take three deep, slow breaths, and open your eyes when you are ready.

www.GenevaMontano.com/WisdomFromTheWomb

***

WISDOM FROM THE WOMB

WHAT DOES IT MEAN to have a baby-led birth?

In the busy lives we all lead in the 21st century, where most pregnant people are working full time in addition to growing a new human, and often raising other children as well, listening to your unborn baby might sound like crazy talk. We are generally taught to listen to our care providers— care providers who might recommend things like: take your vitamins, go to prenatal appointments, don't gain too much weight, and make sure you make it to the hospital on time.

These may be important things to do. But it seems many pregnant people are left feeling like something is lacking, that a piece of their care is missing. They might not be able to put their finger on what exactly it is they had hoped their prenatal care might look like, but they sense they are not getting it at their doctor's office.

I propose that what is missing is a true connection with the baby.

In an effort to remedy the connection missing between baby and parent, our culture bombards us with things like elaborate baby showers, genetic testing, 4D ultrasounds, and gender reveal parties. We think, if we can buy enough things for the baby or create the perfect-themed nursery or see what their face looks like, somehow we will feel better about what our subconscious minds know is missing—a true connection to this new human.

I can't think of any pregnant person I know who felt more at peace about their upcoming birth experience because they had the perfect cake at their baby shower. The sense of community support people long for is rarely fulfilled by the plethora of pink pajamas they are gifted.

While genetic testing and ultrasounds can be both interesting and important for some people, they do not usually create less stress for families. Pregnant people will always find something to worry about—it has been said that worry is the work of pregnancy. If every test and scan come back perfect, the pregnancy will not likely continue without a care. And if every test does not come back perfect, parents endure many months of deep stress that may or may not be warranted, before the baby is Earth-side.

In the intimate dance of pregnancy and childbirth, there are two partners: the person carrying the baby and the baby itself. During pregnancy, our culture focuses mostly on the physical state of the person carrying the baby. We make sure there are no problems arising. We test their blood and their urine; we measure their uterus and their pelvis. We check their blood pressure, their blood sugar and their genetic makeup. Rarely is the spiritual, emotional, or mental state of the baby-carrier addressed, unless it is drastically affecting one of the aforementioned physical aspects.

The true nature and spirit of the baby is not a big part of prenatal care. We may measure their heart rate and sometimes their head circumference, femur length, and amniotic fluid index, while we also try to see what's between their legs. But who this tiny human might be or how they feel is given very little thought. After the birth everything shifts and the baby becomes the full focus of attention, while we start to almost completely ignore the person who just birthed it.

Both the baby carrier and the baby are far more complex beings than modern day prenatal care addresses. The physical is a critically important piece of care. But as holistic beings, our emotional and spiritual health and our physical health are directly impacted by each other. This is true for the parent, but it is also true for the baby, even while they are still in utero.

Your baby is already a person, even before they're born. There has been decades of research that shows babies are reactive to their environment in the womb. They startle when there are loud noises or a rush of adrenaline. Fetal eyes are fused until around 26 weeks, yet ultrasound images have shown babies moving away from needles placed into the uterus or sometimes grabbing the needles. Without even seeing it, a baby senses a trespasser in its watery world and tries to interact with it in some way. Babies' brain waves have shown they feel pain and stress.

We have very little understanding of the fetal world, but the more we learn, the more we know that babies are very complex humans with a wide range of emotions. Their perfect, tiny bodies are still trying to figure out how to maneuver in this physical world, but their minds, especially the parts that control the feeling of safety and emotional intelligence, are fully functioning. They may not yet be thinking the way we as adults are filled with incessant thoughts. But they know a great deal, and they definitely react to their environment.

We have evidence that every memory, starting in utero,

is stored somewhere in the brain; most of us just don't know how to access these memories as adults.[1] Through hypnosis, guided meditation, and other psychotherapy, some people vividly remember birth, the time in utero, and how they felt during those times. Your baby is already a person with feelings and the ability to feel, remember, and communicate.

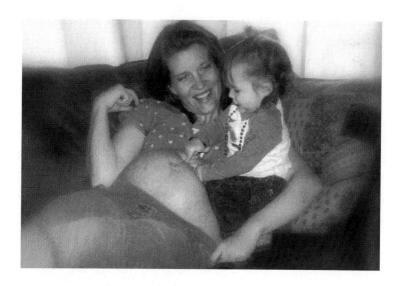

My dear friend Whitney, tells a story about her son, Ember. Ember's birth was quick and hard, and at the end he struggled to get out. His shoulders got stuck, and he inhaled some of the meconium—the baby's first bowel movement. She also got an unwanted and unconsented episiotomy.

His entire early life, Ember was afraid of many things. He didn't like going to the playground; he was clingy and needed a lot of support and encouragement from his parents. When he was about three years old, Whitney pulled him onto her lap and asked him if he remembered his birth.

He said no.

Whitney said, "Well I do, and it was pretty scary."

Ember replied, "Yeah, I couldn't breathe."

Whitney talked to him more about her experience of the birth and how she did her best to keep him safe, and that now, in his big-boy body, he was safe, he could breathe. Later that day, Ember went down the slide at the park for the first time. The memory of his birth was affecting his childhood in ways no one might have imagined.

I have to believe we all have these types of memories that affect us in real ways, whether we choose to acknowledge them or are consciously aware of it or not.

***

I believe your baby is an infinite soul that has lived many previous lifetimes and has now chosen specifically to be incarnated in this time and place and specifically to be carried by you, in your womb. I believe each soul picks its parents—that it searches to find the perfect people who will come together to create the unique learning experiences this soul needs and wants to experience during this lifetime.

Your baby is a cosmic being who has decided that a human experience will offer a benefit to them and has chosen to enter this dimension through the fusing of an egg and a sperm. There is already a plan for what they want to learn and teach during their life here. This begins from the time in utero, before their birth. From an unconfined perspective prior to conception, outside this finite lifetime, a soul has the ability to see each human's ancestral line, the things that have been written in their DNA, their genetics and epigenetics, the environment in which the soul will be gestated, the hormones that will bathe their cells as they grow in a particular womb. They chose exactly the right womb for the experience they desire to have. What if babies know exactly how their birth needs to be, in order to live their best life and bring the highest good to humanity? I wonder how our perceptions of ourselves as birth-givers, and as parents would shift, if we truly believed these fresh souls, these babies, know more about what is needed than we do. I believe babies know a lot more than we give them credit for.

They do not have the years of trauma and distraction we have had as adults. It is said we spend our adult lives trying to heal the wounds that were inflicted during our first six years of life. Your baby has not experienced this wounding yet. They have not forgotten or become distracted from their purpose. As adults, it is easy for us to forget, through all the trauma and distraction, how to trust ourselves. We forget who we are and that we are powerful creators. We forget that trusting ourselves, our guts, our intuitions, is even a possibility! But babies... they remember! They know exactly what it is they are here for. Every cell of their bodies is still in complete knowing and trust that they have come into this lifetime for a purpose.

This belief might seem far-fetched to some people. There might be people who cannot wrap their minds around a soul choosing its parents or knowing what will happen before birth. If this is you, maybe you can stick with me and still agree that the fetus, at some point, is or becomes a sentient being?

The point in time this happens varies in different belief systems. Science has, as of yet, been unable to pinpoint the exact moment life begins. Everyone in the US understands that the question of when a fetus starts being defined as a person is a hot topic. Look at the debate between pro-life versus pro-choice. Does life begin at conception? Or when the heart beats for the first time? Or some other time?

The Bible tells of God knowing Jeremiah before he was in his mother's womb. Some cultures believe the soul drops into the baby when the baby drops in the pelvis. Some have a ceremony at seven months gestation. New technology has been able to record a flash of energy as the sperm and egg unite. No matter when the exact moment of life begins, it seems most people can agree that at some point an unborn baby is indeed alive and already a person. Therefore, they have a will of their own and thoughts and feelings of their own. If you have a baby in your body, or have ever had a baby in your body, you can feel the truth in your spirit that this being inside of you is its own person—an individual with its own life force that is connected to you but possesses a will outside of your own.

Part of the definition of a sentient being is the ability to communicate. Just because the baby does not "talk" does not mean they cannot communicate. It is a well-known fact that most communication from human to human does not just consist of spoken words, but of an intricate system of body language, inflection, underlying nuances, feelings, and more. Pets cannot talk, and yet they communicate clearly with their owners. Science has discovered that trees have a silent and not fully understood but concrete way of communicating with each other.

When we travel to a different country, we may not speak the same language, yet we can almost always convey our needs and wants to those around us. We can sense the emotions and needs of people around us without their speaking. When two people really know each other, they can connect and communicate to one another's hearts and spirits from across the world without a word ever being spoken.

Our babies communicate with us, too. We have simply forgotten how to listen. We sometimes talk to our babies. We tell them that we love them, tell them what to do and how to do it, tell them what their life is going to be like... But rarely do we listen.

What if we, as birthing people, could lean into the trust and wisdom of the baby? If we really listen, can we hear what the baby wants? Can we hear a bigger, divine purpose instead of what we, in our limited view of the present moment, think the plan should be? Would it be possible to make decisions about the pregnancy and the birth based on a pause... a pause where we tune in and listen to something inside of us? Where we learn to talk to our babies and then listen—actually listen—to what the baby has to tell us.

This might seem crazy to the logical mind of a 21st-century American. But can it be any crazier than a world where a third of babies are born surgically and are placed immediately on a machine instead of into the arms of a loving parent? Where a third of women have mood disorders related to pregnancy and birth? Where most people you encounter as a pregnant person hated birth so much that they are willing to tell a stranger to just "get the drugs" or "cut the baby out" as quickly as possible, in order to spare others the fear, pain, and trauma they felt.

When these situations are seen as normal, we have lost something. Many people feel disconnected after birth. Lost or alone—often leading to anxiety, depression, and difficulty parenting. I believe a true connection to our babies on the inside could help bring us to a place of trusting our bodies, our births, and ourselves as parents. This type of trust can lead to healthier families, communities, and societies.

You can ask anyone who has had a baby or who works in the birth field: the birthing person is not really in control of their birth. It does not matter what amount of planning or preparing or self-educating a parent has done, they cannot control what happens during their birth. You cannot ever know enough to keep yourself from having a cesarean birth. You cannot ever do enough positioning in pregnancy and labor to guarantee an efficient birth. You cannot take the right medicine or herbs and make your baby come before their birthday. No one has ever magically checked all the right boxes and *poof!* Had the exact birth that they planned. Even if it was positive and amazing—not everything went exactly as planned.

Maybe this is because the baby is in charge. In the dance of birth, the baby is leading, and the person carrying the baby has to learn to listen to the subtle cues the baby is giving and gracefully follow. In this day and age, a care provider's protocols also impact this dance. They provide the structure within which the baby can guide the dance—the boundaries or the dance floor, if you will. But ultimately, the baby has control.

This takes a lot of pressure off! You don't have to learn everything about birth! You don't have to wear yourself out in labor, trying to know all the right positions or techniques to try. You just have to tune in to your baby and let them guide you through the process. Trust they know what is best in this experience and whatever happens, it was always the plan.

You are an important part of the dance! Your wishes matter! Tell your baby about the things you hope and desire. Create a relationship with this person growing inside you! I believe your baby will listen to you. You still might not ever be able to fully control how things go.

How might your experience feel if, instead of planning, you went inside to connect with your baby? If you could just listen and trust?

I definitely did not feel I was an expert at listening and trusting with any of my four children, though I do know my babies picked their births, and we had a strong connection prenatally. I loved and trusted them implicitly, without knowing this was what I was doing.

I am still learning, in uncomfortable moments, to remind myself and birthing families how powerful and wise their babies are. Sometimes it feels like a risk to say I believe the baby will communicate with them and the baby is in control, that they can just let go and enjoy. I know my beliefs are not mainstream, and it feels scary to be seen as a quack! Ultimately, I have chosen to follow the path shown to me in life, even when it feels scary. Because, just like in birth, the twists and turns of the journey seem to be more peaceful when I follow, than when I attempt to lead.

When I asked my high self, my guides, God, what specifically I should write about in this book about birth, which is my passion and my calling, the answer I received was, "Listen to the baby."

I went to see Abraham and Esther Hicks Live, and the message I walked away with was also that we need to listen to babies. It's interesting because I have listened to hundreds of hours of Abraham Hicks recordings over the years, and I don't actually remember ever hearing them talk about babies. Ever.

(Esther Hicks is a woman who channels a group of spirits called Abraham. Their teachings, to me, seem raw and true, devoid of any fluff or dogma, just universal truth, like the teachings of Jesus. They are some of the original teachers of the law of attraction, amongst other things.)

So, I believe I am meant to share this message: in the birth culture of America in the twenty-first century, we are forgetting that there is another being involved in this process. We have to remember these conscious beings, our babies, and include them in the process. Listen to their wisdom. Allow them to guide their own birth.

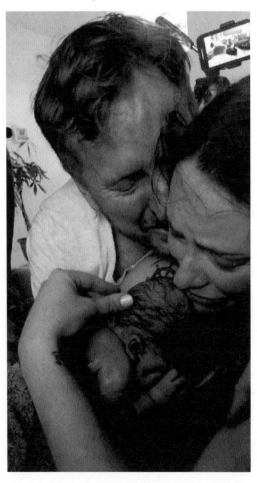

***

In the midwifery world, we talk about there being baby midwives and mom midwives. How each midwife is generally drawn to the work either for the babies or for the birthing people. I myself have always considered myself a mom midwife. I love seeing pregnant people go through their journey and the changes that happen in their life.

Birth is a rite of passage for female-bodied people and has been throughout time. It is a sacred time, and magical things happen during pregnancy, birth, and the early postpartum period. Things that create cracks and scars as they grow and change people for the rest of their lives. I find these scars to be so beautiful. Like the tiny cracks in antique porcelain or the tiger-claw stretch marks on a belly. In pregnancy, birth, and postpartum, women get to touch true joy, true fear, true grief, true intimacy in ways that are otherwise untouchable. The cracks and scars are the places where the light shines through.

Don't get me wrong, I love babies! I'm just not a midwife who does this work for the love of babies. But I do trust them.

I trust with all my being that what happens in each birth is precisely what that baby needs, even when the experience is heartbreakingly confusing to the parents. These babies, when we are still and quiet, can teach us so much.

I am always amazed at how unique, how fully formed, how wise, and how powerful each baby is. How they are already fully themselves at the moment of birth. Each one has a completely unique personality, as different as the swirls in their footprints. And what I realize more and more, as I remember birth stories and continue to work with parents who trust their babies, is that births go smoothest, families are happiest, when the baby is allowed to lead.

I remember my own first baby. When he was born, he was so quiet and curious. He looked around, taking everything in, and had such wisdom and understanding in his silent eyes. It was as if he expected to see the things he saw and was just confirming his knowing.

He never once seemed surprised at the new world all around him, and this surprised me! I expected him to look confused in some way—to seem lost or new in this world. But he did not. I felt in my gut that everything he had experienced was exactly what he'd expected.

I believe this knowing was with him in utero. That he knew what was going to happen; he knew what he needed, knew he would go through the process of being born, and knew what was waiting for him. Maybe he even knew what to expect more than I did, since he did not have the distractions of this Earth-side life, like I had.

So back to the original question: what does it mean to have a baby led birth? How can we listen to someone who is trapped in a uterus and doesn't make sound?

And the answer is (insert drum roll) ...

I don't know.

I do not know exactly how you, personally, will tune in to listen to your baby. I can't tell you how to do this. But I believe you know. As a pregnant person, you have a unique and miraculous connection to the amazing being growing within your body. And you can discover the ways you hear or feel, or imagine or experience your baby.

Maybe your baby will come to you in your dreams. Maybe you will hear a still, small voice and understand it is your baby. Maybe your baby will show you visions or actual physical symbols or signs that you know come from them. Maybe you will meditate or journal and learn to connect with your baby and have conversations with them in those times. Maybe through movement you will feel in your body what your baby needs you to feel. Maybe you will draw or create images that your baby uses to communicate.

People receive the wisdom of babies in different ways, so you will need to find the ways and the words and the imagery that suits and supports you best. I believe that your baby has a purpose and can communicate that purpose with you in their own unique and real way.

However, this book can still be a useful guide for you, even if you do not believe that. When I refer to listening to your baby, you could replace those words with trusting God, Jesus, Mother Nature, or the universe; trusting your guides, your ancestors, your angels, your higher self, your intuition; or listening to your own powerful body—whatever it is that speaks to your heart and your power centers. Only you know who or what you can trust to guide you. This is not something anyone can teach you or tell you how to do.

What is necessary is dedicated quiet time. It will require you to set aside time every day to be still and connect with your baby. This is a non-negotiable. I know you are busy. If you have other children, it is hard to find quiet time alone. If you have a job or career, it certainly takes up many hours in your day. You are probably tired; building and growing a baby takes a lot of energy. But this is important, and I know, if you just decide to make it a priority, you will find the time. The time will manifest even when you previously thought you didn't have it.

Your baby does not understand clocks. They still live

outside of time as you and I understand it. They sleep when they are tired, and they have a continuous flow of nutrients. Their pacing is far slower than ours. Bringing their little fingers to their mouth is a process that can take minutes. There is no rush. There is no deadline and no finish line. You have to understand this pacing in order to connect with your baby.

Slow. Down.

Place a hand on your uterus and breathe into your baby. Just breathe. Allow your breath to sink into a timeless fetal pacing. Just breathe and be open to connecting to your baby. No expectations, no rush. Just breathing and listening.

Slow.

Even slower.

This slow, long pause is the key to listening to your baby.

If you are not accustomed to taking quiet time in your day, it might take a few days, even a few weeks of daily practice, for you to feel confident that you are hearing your baby's still, small whispers.

You might feel crazy at first, when you start to believe you are hearing your baby. That's okay! It takes practice to trust your baby, and every time you do it, you will get better at it, and it will help you through your birth and through parenting. I promise, the more you do it, the easier it becomes.

Commit to slowing down and trying to connect for twenty minutes, twice a day, for a week. (If twenty minutes seems impossible, try five minutes, two minutes—heck, even twenty seconds! Just commit to taking time.)

First thing in the morning and right before bed are great times, but there is no wrong time to do it. I am willing to bet, if you stop after that week, you will realize that you miss your baby. You miss the time you got to spend with them. This should not be a chore—it is a privilege to be so close to another being. This is the closest you will ever be to anyone in your life! Enjoy it!

I offer many different practices throughout this book to help you connect. Remember: they are practices! Meaning, you will get more out of them the more often and regularly you do them, and you are not ever expected to do them perfectly.

Some of them might seem weird. You might notice your mind wander during some of them. If your baby starts to guide you into a different practice, like one of the ideas mentioned above or something else, follow that! Trust you will know exactly how your baby wants to communicate with you. Just remember: it will be slow and hushed, never rushed, like swimming through honey. Delicious and sweet. But slow and sticky.

Can you be open to the knowing that your baby will guide you through your pregnancy? Through the process of birth? Through the trying times of deciphering postpartum and infancy?

My hope is you will just remain open and commit to making the time to connect with your baby. As I share some of the wisdom and stories I have gleaned over the past fifteen years of birth work, I hope you can remain in the knowing that I am not an expert on your birth. But *you* are, and your baby is. You already have everything you need to have the best possible birth experience. You have a miraculously strong body, a fetus who is a powerful, creative, pristine being, and an opportunity to pause, grow quiet, and listen to the wisdom from your womb.

***

Womb Connection
Practice Listening

* Find a quiet space. If it helps you to put on gentle music or shamanic drumming, please do so. You can lie down or sit on a cushion with your spine straight and your heart open.

* Place one hand on your heart and the other on your baby. Notice your breath. As thoughts come to your mind, notice those as well, but come back to your breath.

* Ask your baby how you can most easily connect to them today. In what way will you hear their voice strongest today. Continue asking this question for a few minutes. You may receive an answer immediately; you may not.

* When you receive communication from your baby, it is like a flash. You don't have to think about it, weigh the pros and cons, or sit and wonder if that is your baby talking. If you get a flash of information, just trust it, and try to connect in whatever way was given to you...

* When you receive that flash of an answer, please continue connecting with your baby in whatever way you heard would be best. Honor the baby's answer immediately.

If you did not hear an answer, be open for the rest of the day to receiving one. Every time you feel your baby kick, let it be a reminder to you that they are communicating with you, and ask them how you can most easily connect today.

* Each time you have to make a decision, see if you can quickly check in with baby and see if they have any input.

* Pay attention to words other people say to you, you hear in music, or you see around you on signs or anywhere else.

* Before you go to bed, remind your baby you are waiting for an answer, and see if the answer comes in your dreams.

Just start practicing. It might feel weird and that's okay. Be slow. Find time. Trust. Your baby is communicating with you, and you are learning how to listen. It will get easier with practice.

www.GenevaMontano.com/WisdomFromTheWomb

***

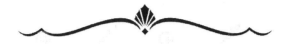

Womb Wisdom:
Caroline's Story

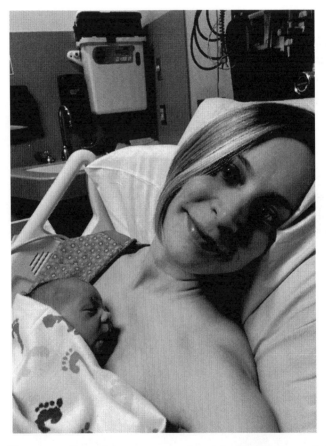

Caroline transferred to my care about halfway through her first pregnancy. She has such a sweet, unassuming spirit, and she cries when she talks about things that touch her heart, which is just about everything. Her vulnerability is captivating.

Throughout her pregnancy, we were unsure about her baby's position. We had deep conversations about the trust she had in her baby, Olivia. She taught me so much about what it means to live in the space of trusting the baby. Each time a decision needed to be made, I saw her check in with Olivia.

One time when we were talking about Caroline's own birth, Caroline revealed through teary eyes that she was born by cesarean because she was breech, and when she explored her own birth, she felt like her mother didn't trust her. She said she had carried this feeling with her even into adulthood. She was worried about telling her parents she had decided to have a home birth, because she didn't think her parents trusted her to make the best decision for her family.

Olivia was also breech early on, but we thought maybe she had turned head down in the third trimester. Around 36 weeks, I asked Caroline to get an ultrasound to make sure, and it turned out she was still breech. Caroline took every measure in the book to get Olivia to turn. She did acupuncture, chiropractic, pelvic tilts, all the spinning-babies techniques. She talked to her baby, and she had her husband, Nick, talk to her baby.

We went to see an OB to attempt an external version, and Olivia did not enjoy that experience. She had some decelerations in her heart rate, and it was scary. It was scary for me, and it was scary for Nick and Caroline. I can only imagine how Olivia felt. So, we went to Plan C.

There is one hospital in our area that offers vaginal breech birth, so we called them to schedule a consult visit, to see if Caroline would be a good candidate for vaginal breech. They often only allow second-time moms to attempt vaginal breech birth, but we figured it was worth a shot. I had worked with another family earlier that month who had a successful vaginal breech birth at the same hospital, and she was also a first-time mom, so I knew there was a chance.

Caroline and I had several more conversations about her options, and the theme of each of them was trusting her baby and checking in to see what Olivia wanted to do.

Caroline went into labor the night before her consult visit. She had mild contractions throughout the day that strengthened around bedtime. A couple hours later, her water broke, and a couple hours after that, they asked me to come to their home. The plan was to labor at home as long as possible and head to the hospital to deliver the baby.

When I arrived at her home, she was having strong contractions. I checked her cervix, and she was only 2 cm, so I encouraged them to tuck in and sleep for a little while longer, and I went downstairs and tucked myself into their guest bed.

About forty minutes later, to my surprise I heard the unmistakable sound of a mom getting close to pushing. I went upstairs and saw Caroline trying to crawl somewhere. It looked like maybe she was trying to crawl away from her own body! We decided it was a good time to go to the hospital.

On arrival, she was already completely dilated. The doctor who greeted us was friendly and warm and said, if Caroline wanted to attempt a vaginal breech birth, she was as good a candidate as anyone. What surprised me in this moment was, even though Caroline had had so many conversations with me and with her husband that the vaginal breech was the route she wanted to go, in that moment she closed her eyes, took several breaths and checked in with Olivia before she decided. Olivia still said that she wanted to be born vaginally.

We all went back into the operating room, which Caroline wisely called the pushing room. Nick was overwhelmed with emotion. He was worried about his wife and baby and amazed at how strong she was. Amazed that she could endure such intensity.

The doctors were hands-off and encouraging. And Caroline was brilliant. She gave birth to Olivia after only about thirty minutes of pushing. Olivia was taken to the warmer for resuscitation, which is not uncommon with breech babies, and Caroline never had a doubt that her baby would be fine. She knew she had listened to exactly what Olivia needed throughout pregnancy and throughout the birthing time, and her baby would soon be in her arms.

I am so proud of Caroline, Nick, and Olivia. Caroline's mom came to visit, and she was proud, too. She told Caroline how impressed she was that Caroline had made such wise decisions for herself, her birth, and her baby, and expressed how she wished she had had a chance to make similar decisions when Caroline was born. She said through teary eyes that she was never given any options.

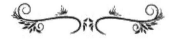

FINDING MY OWN WOMB WISDOM

WHEN I WAS TWENTY-TWO, I got pregnant unexpectedly with my first baby. This may be the first time I realized for certain that I was not in control of my life.

I had a great plan. I had recently graduated from college with a degree in foreign languages. I was very involved in my church and committed to following what I thought the Bible wanted me to do, and as such, I was celibate. I had been to Russia three times as a missionary, and I already had my ticket to move to Siberia in March of 2000, to live and work with the church for two years. I would come back and get my master's degree in inner city ministry in Chicago.

Such a great plan! My twenty-two-year-old self couldn't wait to get going. But in November 1999, I met a guy I had some good chemistry with, we had sex a few times, and my plan was over. My life was forever changed! Instead of going to Russia to be a missionary, I became a mother.

Honestly, it was probably the hardest time in my life. I loved my baby so much, but I felt like an outsider. I felt like I had failed my God and my family, both blood and chosen. I was pregnant by a man I hardly knew. And then I had a baby.

Having a baby for the first time is so isolating for most women in this country, and I was certainly no different. I was alone all day, trying to figure out how to get my baby to stop crying. He cried all the time, especially when we were home alone.

I wasn't upset at him for this, although there were a few moments where I could understand why people get to the point where they would be tempted to shake a baby. I was upset at myself. Why couldn't I figure this out? Why was my life and my house in chaos? Why didn't my baby love me? Why was this so hard? Why wasn't I good enough? I felt completely alone.

My friends went on with their lives. My family loved my baby, but they were all busy with their lives. My baby's dad had just opened a new business, and he was pretty wrapped up in the ins and outs of making it successful. We didn't live together at the time, and I had never really seen an example of a dad who was very involved and confident with his newborn, so I didn't think anything of it that he was too busy to make sure I was okay. And we hardly knew each other anyway, I didn't feel like I could ask him for much.

I didn't feel like I could ask anyone for much. I was the epitome of the woman about whom I warn the families I work with. The woman who won't accept help, who feels like, if she were strong enough, courageous enough, just *enough...* that she would be able to do all these things on her own. So, I laid on the couch while my baby nursed and just drifted in and out of life for a year or so. I lost myself.

The good thing was, I felt really great about my birth. I had a vaginal, unmedicated birth. I thought that was pretty cool. I felt like a badass when I thought about my birth. I looked back at pictures from that day and I was *beautiful.*

Strong. Radiant. I remembered how mesmerizing my baby looked when he came out. His big, round eyes looking around, soaking everything in. I could tell at that moment this baby would be a genius.

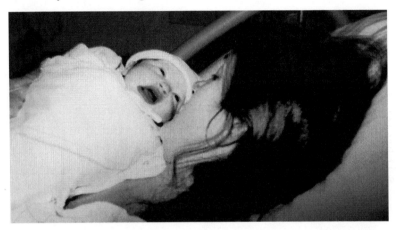

His birth took thirteen hours from the first contraction to holding my baby in my arms. It was probably the most textbook birth I have ever been a part of! I was at a teaching hospital, and the doctor who came in for the birth (whom I had never met until that moment) brought several medical students in with him, because they had never witnessed a natural birth before.

I was never invited to push in a position other than lying on my back while pulling on my knees. When I told the nurse I needed a break, she told me I couldn't have one. But I did it. I pushed that baby out with nothing but my inner fire.

I loved my baby and the beautiful experience my baby allowed me to have. Man, he was cute. He had luscious black curls and the darkest chocolate eyes, with eyelashes that looked like daddy long-legs. He loved to nurse and got so fat, he weighed seventeen pounds at three months! I remember watching him in awe. It was amazing to see him figure out that he could control his hands and then his feet. To see him start to interact with his world, smile, laugh, try to get a reaction from people.

I had honestly never really heard of anyone having a positive birth experience up to that point. I had heard how hard and painful it would be. I had heard I should get the drugs. No one ever told me they felt like a goddess, fierce and full of raw power, that while giving birth they died and came back a new person, even though the world around them couldn't seem to recognize the changes.

It's surreal to experience something so profound and feel like you've been reborn, and somehow expect the world to have shifted with you, but then realize not one thing seems to have changed in anyone else's life but your own. And to sometimes get a little stuck and not know who this new person is or what she needs or how the two of you, the old you and the new you, can share this body, this existence.

I felt I had to find a new path after having my baby. Traveling around the world to spread the gospel no longer seemed like an option with a newborn. I did some student teaching while I was pregnant, because I figured, with a degree in foreign languages, that would be the most logical choice. Turns out you have to really want to be a teacher. It is not for the faint of heart! I tried bookkeeping. I worked at my baby's dad's coffee shop. I did some MLM. I even talked to an Army recruiter. Nothing really spoke to me.

I really wanted to work with the church, so I tried to work with the youth group or teach Sunday School. But the church told me I was not a good example to the teenagers or the children, being an unwed mother and all, so I was not allowed to do that anymore. I was devastated and had no idea who I was or who I was supposed to be.

One day, my best friend, who was a huge lover of birth and pregnancy, and who believed in natural birth even though she had had three cesareans, told me about childbirth educators. She said you could become one without being a nurse, and they made decent money during evening and weekend hours. So, I decided to give it a shot.

***

I say over and over that birth is just like life. Whatever big challenges you can think of that come up in life, an analogy for that challenge comes up in birth. Birth tries to teach us the lessons we have chosen to learn in this lifetime. My life is no different. I believe birth is mostly intuitive, that the baby guides us through the pregnancy and through the birth, and when we learn to listen, a tiny whisper will guide us through our lives as well. I have not always been good at listening to that voice, so the universe often has had to just push me where I needed to go!

Honestly, I have never really felt like I decided to become a birth worker. Becoming a childbirth educator was the first time I was pushed onto the path to where I am now: a midwife. I didn't even know midwives still practiced home birth, when I started my training to be a Lamaze-certified childbirth educator.

I found a book when I was nine months pregnant with my second baby that talked about midwives, and I checked it out from the library and excitedly shared it with my best friend. I had an aha moment that we could be midwives! I told her we could care for women, just like doctors, only with less time in school! I may not have completely understood what this entailed at the time, but the seed was planted.

I have always felt like the universe or God has laid a path

in front of me, and I have somehow just continued fumbling—taking steps, bumping into walls, taking detours, sometimes getting pushed or dragged, but always moving forward on the path that led me to where I am now.

I had my second baby in the hospital with a midwife. I had gotten married the year before, and we were struggling to make ends meet. Every day felt like an uphill battle, but I was immensely proud of my brilliant two-year-old and was committed to creating a perfect little family.

I was really tired during the last days of that pregnancy. Before labor even started, I was already thinking I wasn't sure I had the energy to get through labor, and I certainly manifested that.

My labor was moving really fast, but I didn't know that at the time. I just knew it was really intense. More intense than I remembered the first birth being. I never actually asked for an epidural, but I asked what my pain relief options were, and the next thing I knew, there was an anesthesiologist in my room. Somewhere inside myself I knew I could say no at this point, but it was just so easy *not* to say no! So, I said yes.

My midwife came in while I was getting the epidural and said, "You're already tired?"

I don't know why she said that, but it impacted me greatly. Had she come in five minutes earlier, maybe she could have helped me, and I would have had another unmedicated birth, as I had planned. But instead, I felt shamed by her. I felt like, if I were strong enough, I wouldn't have needed the pain medications and again, like I had failed myself and my baby. I'm not opposed to epidurals. I think they are a great tool for some births. But I didn't think I actually needed one. I just needed something different to happen. The shame I felt from that simple comment affected my belief in myself as a woman, as a mother, as a human.

After I got comfortable, my water broke and my son was born a few minutes later. He had a one-minute APGAR of 2, so he was taken over to the warmer. I didn't get to have immediate skin-to-skin with him, I didn't know if he was okay, and I was scared.

He had the umbilical cord wrapped around his neck, body, and arm. But after he was given a few breaths with the bag-mask to open his lungs and a few minutes to transition to life on Earth, he was doing fine, and they brought him over to me. I never felt connected to that birth experience. I don't know if it was the pain meds or the fear, but something was different. I still loved my baby, but I felt disconnected. I judged myself harshly for many years, both for the fact that I got an epidural and that I felt distant from the entire experience. I came up against the familiar feeling that I had failed: failed myself, failed my baby, failed the women who had come before me, and those who would come after.

The hospital where my son was born had a one to three-hour mandatory observation period for all babies. So, they took my brand-new son to the nursery and told me to get some rest. My husband's birthday was the day before my son was born, so he asked if he could go to a concert with his friends that night. I had just had a baby two hours prior to this, but it never really occurred to me that I could say no. I still thought I couldn't really ask him, or anyone, for anything. So, again, though I wanted him to stay, I said yes. My mom was at home with my sweet two-year-old.

I was alone. Sometime in the middle of the night, after not sleeping at all, I started getting really antsy, wondering why they didn't bring my baby back. I hit the nurse call button, and no one responded. I wandered around the halls for a few minutes but didn't know where to go in this huge hospital ward, where all the walls and doors looked the same. I still never bothered anyone. I sat alone in my room, worried, scared, lonely, not knowing what I should do.

That was the day I decided I would never have another baby in a hospital. And I didn't know it at the time, but that was the day I decided that no birthing person should ever have to wonder where their baby is or be scared and alone after they'd just pushed a baby out. That was the day my baby whispered to me that I needed to become a warrior for birth.

A year or so after that birth, I was working in my new field, teaching childbirth classes in a hospital, and people started asking me if I would attend their births with them, so I became a doula. Then a position opened up at the hospital, and I started working as a staff doula there. I had the blessing of being able to attend about 150 births there, learning the ins and outs of hospital birth. I really loved teaching classes at the hospital, sharing my passion for birth and for babies with excited new families. It was fun being able to see some of them when they went into labor and be their doula, as well.

After a couple years of teaching and being a hospital doula, witnessing so many births, some in which people were really in their power and some where people had yet to realize how powerful they are, I began looking for ways to become a midwife. I still didn't really even know that home birth was a legitimate option in this country, but somehow, I stumbled upon a website online that offered a two-year course to start training to become a homebirth midwife. Looking back, I can see all along I was just being pushed along the path. Guided.

While I was doing my homebirth courses, I found myself pregnant again. My entire family and husband thought I might be a little crazy, but of course, I had a homebirth. It really never occurred to me to care what anyone else thought about my decision. I knew this baby wanted to be born at home.

During my pregnancy, I experienced several bouts of unexplained bleeding. One of the times, I was at work when it happened, so I walked over to the labor and delivery ward and asked one of the nurses to listen to the baby's heartbeat, just so I could have some reassurance.

She said, "Well, if you are having a miscarriage, there's nothing we can do about it anyway."

And my heart fell. I felt heartbroken for myself, for feeling unsupported, for my baby, that no one cared if she lived or died, and for all women who receive less-than-loving care. I learned during that pregnancy how much we love our babies, not for anything they do or for anything that has to do with their physical existence, but just because we love them. I knew nothing about this brand-new human, and yet I loved her so much and grieved deeply at the thought of losing her. I knew her and wanted her and loved her so much before I ever felt her move or had any sense of the amazing person she would be.

This is true of each one of us. Our spirit, our being, is loved and is pure love in itself, from the moment it decides to incarnate. We are loved simply for our existence. I had to learn to trust pregnancy and birth in a whole new way with my third baby. I never had an ultrasound to give me the sense of security that all was well. I just trusted she was. She was also breech at 38 weeks. Breech birth is illegal at home in my state, so I had to trust that she would turn, so I could have the home birth I knew we both wanted. She did.

Oh, my goodness, I just cannot ever explain the sweetness and magic of home birth. It was the most peaceful, relaxing, and natural experience. The baby just came out. There was no fuss, nothing that needed to be done. It was like it was just supposed to happen... and it did! Such a powerful experience.

Okay—I'm not going to lie. It was still intense. One of the hardest things I've ever done. But my sweet daughter was born in the caul (this means the amniotic sac didn't break until after she was born), undisturbed, without so much as a vaginal exam.

Let me be honest here—I wanted a vaginal exam! When I felt my body pushing, I asked my midwife to check me, and she said that she had no need to check me and wanted to know why I wanted to be checked.

I told her, "Because I don't trust my body!" She chuckled, and a few minutes later my baby was born.

My midwife was adamant I take time to rest and be supported after the birth. I cried when she came over and brought me a casserole and refilled my peri bottle for me. Shout out to my midwife, Sena Johnson, who trusts women's bodies, even when they don't trust themselves, and who believes with her actions as well as her words in women being held and supported after birth.

Luckily, since I loved that experience so much, I got pregnant *again* a few months later! Yes, I had a six-month-old, a five-year-old, and an eight-year-old when I found myself with child yet again. I cried every day for about four months, because I did not know how I could have another baby when I already had a baby. I was unsure whether or not this baby was meant to be.

My best friend and I researched ways to naturally end a pregnancy. I asked my midwife what she recommended. She said that if I really didn't want to be pregnant, I would have to show the universe I was serious about it in some way, and she said she supported me whatever I decided. I asked my husband what he thought we should do. He said he thought I should get an abortion. The moment I heard those words, I felt 100% positive, as sure as I've ever been about anything in my life, that she needed to be born.

I had the easiest pregnancy with her. I think God knew I could not handle anything more than what I was already dealing with. I loved being pregnant with her, and I was sad when I went into labor ten days before my due date. I was actually so in denial that she was coming, I drove myself across the city to my prenatal appointment and back while I was in labor. She was born ninety minutes after I got home.

It was another beautiful home birth, surrounded by my children. Fast and hard. And magical and peaceful. My midwife, Sena, told me I made birth look easy, and I made her promise she would never say that to anyone again. It was not easy, no matter how it looked. I'm not sure it ever is.

My husband and I were certain this baby would be a boy, so we didn't pick out any girl names. She didn't have a name until she was three days old, when I swear, she told me her name in the middle of the night. It was a name I had never even heard or seen before. We named her Melea, which means "dear friend."

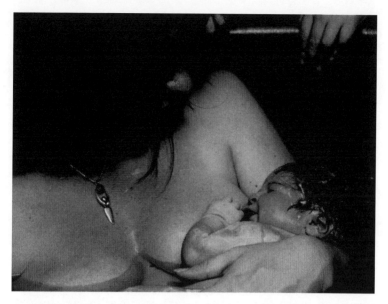

Well, at this point I had four kids, two babies and two I was homeschooling. I was still teaching at the hospital and doing birth and postpartum doula work. My husband was still trying to get his business to be successful. Then an opportunity to work as an apprentice with my midwife opened up! Well, of course, with everything else I had going on, I decided that this was the perfect time to work for free and finish up my midwifery training!

Looking back, I feel like I must have been insane! But I was so excited for this opportunity and could not imagine waiting for another second to start my apprenticeship. So, for about a year and a half, I somehow worked forty hours a week, homeschooled, and apprenticed as a midwife, attending prenatal appointments and several births a month with my preceptor. Until I lost my ever-loving mind.

My marriage was struggling, and all I ever did was yell at my kids. I felt like I was failing at everything I was doing. I missed a couple of doula births, which meant I didn't get paid on top of feeling like I was letting people down left and right. My kids were suffering, being dropped off at random strangers' houses when I had to go to a birth or a prenatal. I was exhausted; I'm not sure if I ever slept. I loved birth work, but I could not really imagine being any less happy in my life, in general. So, I quit.

I decided I should just go to nursing school and become a hospital-based midwife. Something with a schedule that had some consistency to it. I started school for this. I put my kids into public school. The path I had been following felt too hard. It felt like a mountain that was impossible to climb. So, I decided to create my own path, make my own decisions.

Well... even though school was easier than apprenticing and I had more time with my family, it didn't take long to realize it wasn't actually the path to being a midwife that made me miserable. I was just miserable. Life as a parent was hard, and my relationship with my partner was even harder. I had left my church. I was completely focused on taking care of everyone around me, and I was so incredibly lonely. I didn't know who I was.

After a few really difficult hospital doula births, I remembered why I never wanted to be a hospital midwife, and I remembered that bright spot home births brought to my life. So, I started my search to find a new preceptor to finish my training with.

I was blessed to study under several amazing midwives. Midwifery is something you can really only learn by doing and watching, and I am so grateful for the midwives who were gracious enough to share their wisdom and skill with me and, really, their lives as well. Being in an apprentice/preceptor relationship is a lot like a marriage.

You see each other at your best and your worst. I am also grateful that the opportunities to study under the right people were always, *always* placed in my path at the right time. So many people who want to be midwives struggle to find a midwife to study with. I was always placed exactly where I needed to be.

Fast forward a few years and a couple hundred births later and I was a real, legit midwife. I was also divorced, now a happier, single mom of four. I had worked in a partnership with my second preceptor for about a year when I realized the kind of midwifery we were practicing was *not* what I thought midwifery would be. We had good relationships with our clients and gave them high-quality care. But somehow, the magic I'd felt about midwifery was missing.

Somewhere in my heart's ancient wisdom, I knew a midwife is more than just someone who keeps birth safe. She is a healer. A medicine woman. A witch. A shaman. And a trusted friend. Even though I left the church, I have always been a deep and spiritual person and spent my free time learning about healing and God and the magic in our spirits. I realized these two facets of myself could no longer live apart from one another, and I was being called to be a different kind of midwife.

I went to India in November 2017, and I had a vision, a download of what my practice was supposed to look like. I would build community, offer healing work in addition to midwifery care, create sacred space during the birth, and remind women and families how magical and powerful their bodies and their babies are. I would help women listen to their babies. We would build real relationships and laugh and cry together as we support one another. My practice would work on a sliding scale, because money should not be a limiting factor to a baby being born where and how they want to be.

I had a plan to continue working with my then-partner until May 2018, and then start my new solo practice. Turns out my partner didn't think that was the best idea. On January 2, she asked me to leave the keys to the office and return my equipment.

That was a pretty hard push, universe. That one hurt. I was terrified. From one day to the next, I went from having this amazing plan to having nothing. No equipment, no births, no support. I went and got my substitute teaching license, because I had no faith I could be successful as a midwife in a short amount of time, or really that my vision could become a reality at all. Every time I have had a plan, things have gone pretty awry. My life, like birth, seems to work better when I let it unfold in front of me, listening to the quiet voices, rather than making a plan.

***

The great thing about the universe is, when it pushes you, it will always catch you. I don't honestly know where or how families have found me. When I ask, they often don't seem to know either. But you guys, I have had the best people come into my life! I could not imagine having more perfect clients who believe in themselves, believe in birth, believe in me. They trust their babies in a way I could never have imagined. They teach me so much with every birth, every appointment we have. Together we have danced, meditated, shared, laughed, cried, died, and been born again.

My midwifery practice is flourishing. Since 2018, I also became a yoga teacher and completed several other potent healing courses related to birth and life. I trust God and my guides in a way I never have before, and I can see how this path has led me to this present moment. I see how every birth is held, supported, guided by the small voices, the baby, the birthing bodies.

At one birth, there was a "spiritual doula" present, and she told me she could see hundreds of baby spirits around me, that they support me and guide me as a midwife. I feel them and am grateful they chose me.

People in my practice have gotten to know one another, supported one another, formed real community. They have experienced healing—through their births, through divine energy flowing through my hands, through the loving energy of other families, and most especially through these beautiful spirits who have chosen them to be their parents.

My hope is each person I come in contact with can feel the certainty that everything that happens in their pregnancy and birth is divinely guided, and that their babies know the plan, even when they themselves do not. It is beautiful to see the vision I had in India being birthed in my practice. It is beautiful to witness birthing people who truly trust their babies and who are guided through the pregnancy and birthing experience by the communication they have with their babies.

I am still learning what this means and what it looks like. I am taught as I go, and I'm still listening to the babies, just as their parents are. I hope my story and those of the babies I have worked with will bring peace and joy to more families as we explore the birthing journey together and learn to listen to the wisdom from the womb.

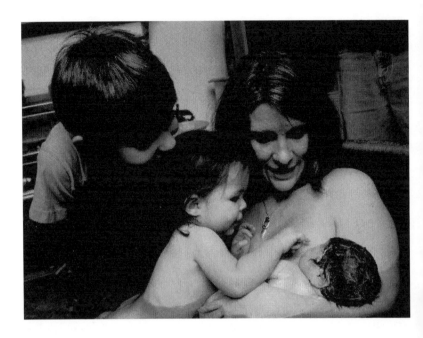

WOMB CONNECTION
WHAT DID YOUR BIRTH STORIES TEACH YOU?

* If you have given birth before, spend some time writing out your own birth story or stories. Notice the places in the story where you feel a lot of energy. What did your baby want you to learn during those highly charged times? Spend some time with your emotions, and see if you can get down to the bottom of the lessons.

For me, in the first birth, I learned my own strength. The second birth, I realized I needed to find my voice. The third birth, I learned to trust. The fourth birth, I learned to give up control.

* If you have not given birth before, ask some of your close friends or family members about their birth experiences. Listen in a way you haven't before. Listen for the lessons that are in their experiences for them and for you. Ask the hard questions that come up, even if it feels uncomfortable.

* What did birth teach them about life and about themselves? How did birth change them? What does your baby want you to learn about yourself through the stories you hear?

www.Genevamontano.com/WisdomFromTheWomb

***

SEEING CYCLES

IF YOU'VE DONE ANY amount of self-help or spiritual growth work in your life, then you know that noticing the cycles in your life is one of the first steps in healing.

Almost everything in our world is based on cycles. Our bodies, the seasons, sleeping, eating, working... You get the point. Women are especially cyclical—our hormones, our own growth and death cycles, and those of the lives created within the womb. Like the moon, we have a period of waxing and waning each month. Start to notice your own cycles and the cycles around you. How do you feel at different points of the cycles in your body or in the world around you—the moon phases or the seasons? What are your daily routines? And what happens if there is a change in these routines? What happens to the Earth when cycles get interrupted?

We don't usually notice the regular rhythms of our lives, because they are so familiar to us. The particular way you do seemingly mundane things is probably a combination of how you learned things from your caregivers and doing things the same way or purposely doing them a different way, plus some social or cultural guidance, plus maybe the influence of the way your partner or other people who are often in your intimate spaces do things.

It can be helpful to really become aware of yourself and why you do things. This can help you determine what things are harmful or helpful to you during your pregnancy and your birthing time, as well as for parenting. Cycles and patterns are natural and useful. They keep us healthy and safe. Sometimes we get stuck in old patterns that are no longer useful. For example, if you grew up in Alaska, you might have a pattern of putting on layers of really warm clothes every day. However, if as an adult you move to Arizona and continue this, a pattern that once served you could begin to harm you.

I encourage you to start paying attention to your own simple cycles and patterns. Notice your thoughts, what you eat, how you make decisions. Pay attention to the way you react to certain situations and be curious about why. Notice your routines, and just be curious about why you do things the way you do. No judgment, just curiosity. Noticing is the first step to finding healing.

***

Womb Connection
Noticing Cycles

✴ Think about your morning routine. What steps do
   you routinely take every day? When did you start
   doing these things? Who taught you? Do these
   things serve you? What happens if you don't do these
   things?

✴ Go a little deeper and think about something you
   don't want to pass on to your baby from your family.
   Who has these traits that you hope your baby will
   avoid? Where did this trait start? What would
   happen if the cycle was interrupted? What would
   replace this trait in your ideal world? What cycles,
   traditions, traits do you hope to pass on to your
   baby?

✴ Now think about your pregnancy and birth. What
   cycles or routines have you brought into pregnancy
   that may or may not resonate? What negative
   emotions come up for you when you think about
   birth that could be the result of a cycle you could
   choose to end? How can your connection to baby
   help begin a new cycle?

www.Genevamontano.com/WisdomFromTheWomb

***

FEAR-TENSION-PAIN CYCLE

There is a deep need to find healing for the birthing experience in the United States. Whether they realize it or not, many people who give birth in this country are experiencing harm physically, mentally, or emotionally. In order to heal this, we have to notice how things are happening: the routine steps and procedures that are taken, and the reasons why we do the things the way we do. We have to notice how and why we react certain ways during pregnancy and birth and be curious about why.

The *Fear-Tension-Pain* cycle is not unique to birth, as all humans experience it at certain points in their life. However, we do sometimes see this cycle spin out of control during the birthing process. In our human experience, when we feel fear, one of the natural responses to that fear in the physical body is to tense up or feel anxious. When we are tense and anxious, that creates a sense of pain in the body. And when we feel pain, most people start to feel fear, wondering if they are okay, if there is something bad happening in their bodies, maybe even if they are dying. And thus, the cycle begins again.

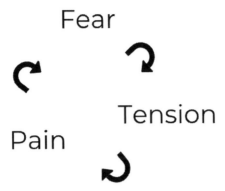

Fear

Tension

Pain

Ideally, we can interrupt this cycle during the birthing process. Perhaps we can replace tension and anxiety with relaxation. In my experience, how well a birthing person can relax during their birthing time is key to how everything else goes. It does not seem to matter whether the birth is long or short, hospital or home, vaginal or cesarean: if the birthing person knows how to get themselves into a state of relaxation, things just seem to go smoother. This, of course, is easier said than done. Most people, will not just go into labor and be in the most Zen state they've ever been in. In fact, most people, do exactly the opposite. They tense up against the intensity of the contractions, or waves, as some midwives call them.

Waves are a great analogy in this particular scenario. If you've ever been in the ocean, you know, if you try to stand tall and strong and rigid against the force of the waves as they crash, you are likely to be knocked down. However, if you relax and float through the waves, you are held by the water as the forceful waves take you for a ride. This is also true in birth. The waves are incredibly powerful, and when we learn to surrender to that power and feel held while the uterus does what it is designed to do, it is a far more enjoyable experience.

Yes, I said it: birth can be *enjoyable* if we can learn to relax around the intensity happening in the uterus.

So, how do you relax while every two to ten minutes you are feeling one of the most intense sensations you have ever felt? It is certainly not easy. But I would argue it is easier to figure out how to relax than it is to have a birth where you don't figure it out. Finding the answer to this question will be one of the most important things for every birthing person to do.

Start trying different ways of relaxing and practicing prenatally. Being connected to your baby and trusting that all is how it is intended to be, is the first step to feeling relaxed. What else works for you? Water? Massage? Scent? Movement? Hypnosis? Somewhere inside yourself, you already know exactly how to relax into your birth.

This wisdom is and has always been in your womb. Clear out the muck that is telling you that you don't know by turning your eyes inward, downward, into your womb. Your contractions cannot be stronger than you. All that power, all the intensity, is created by *you*! It cannot be bigger than you because it is just your uterus contracting. Even if your birth is not vaginal or you never have a single contraction, you still have everything you need within yourself to know how to relax into the experience, whatever it may be. Let's figure this out.

Connecting with your baby will be a huge part of this. Your baby can teach you how to relax. Have you ever spent time with a newborn? All they want to do is relax into a feeling of safety. They eat so they can relax, they poop so that they can relax, they cry only when something is keeping them from being relaxed. Your baby is an expert in letting things go and trusting that all is well.

Tune into that energy from your baby every time you start to feel fear. Even as you read this book, when you start to notice something has triggered you or you are holding tension somewhere in your body, place one or both hands on your belly. Take a breath and feel the connection between you and your baby. Is your baby tense? Are they holding on to anything that is not serving them? Nope. When you feel your baby is relaxed and at ease, take a few breaths and let your baby's state of being melt your tension away.

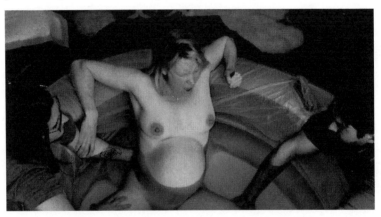

You will replace tension with relaxation. (You can do this; we will continue to figure it out, together with your baby.) Next we also want to replace the fear. Fear is rampant in our culture and, of course, many birthing people have never heard anything about birth that is not steeped in fear.

Before I had my first baby, I had never heard of anyone having a positive birth experience. I'd only heard about how painful it would be, how I should get drugs, how hard the recovery would be, and mostly, that I should do whatever it takes to just get through it with as little interaction as possible with my body or the baby. To just let the doctors take care of me and take care of the pain.

Unfortunately, it's not just birth that is surrounded by fear in our culture. We are taught from a young age that living in fear keeps us safe. If we are afraid enough, we will take the actions necessary to keep bad things away from us. Locks and bars on our doors and windows keep the bad guys out. Going to church keeps us from going to hell. Giving birth with all the bells and whistles keeps our babies safe. And if we do things differently, we are putting ourselves and our families at risk. Many people in this culture don't ask questions, don't check in with their own heart, their own intuition, let alone their babies, about what might be best for their lives or their births.

The truth is there are many potential things that could change the direction of your birth. You could read every book ever written about birth and still not know every possible way things could become complicated. You could worry every day about something that could go "wrong," and you might not ever find the right thing to worry about! So let go of trying to find something that will go sideways. The things that are going to happen during your baby's birth are the lessons your life wants to teach you and that your baby chose you for specifically.

And despite all the things that could go wrong, in all likelihood, you and your baby will be safe. Humans have been having babies for a very long time—from the beginning of time as we know it! Birth is designed to work, and it almost always does. The great thing about living in the 21st century is, even when things don't work perfectly, we do have the safety net of medical care. And while we may know this on a mind level, what we need in order to interrupt the cycle is to replace fear on a heart level.

When I learned about this cycle fifteen years ago, I was taught we could replace fear with knowledge. That we could learn about our options and educate ourselves enough so we would no longer be afraid of this unknown experience. I now think this is the farthest thing from the truth.

When I had my third baby, after I had become a childbirth educator, a doula, and completed two years of midwifery studies, I took some Advil at the beginning of pregnancy. At some point during my schooling, I had learned that ibuprofen in early pregnancy was linked to anencephaly. (*Anencephaly* is the absence of a major portion of the brain and skull that forms during embryonic development, the result of a neural-tube defect.) So, I spent the rest of that pregnancy certain my baby was going to be born anencephalic.

I would lie in bed with my hands on my belly and try to prepare myself for her to be born and only live a few hours. I never got an ultrasound with that pregnancy, and I never told my midwife or my husband I was worried about it until I was well into my third trimester.

Good news! My baby was born with a fully formed, beautiful skull and brain. Point is—*knowing* more does not always give us less to worry about! In fact, it can just give us more things to obsess over that we didn't even know we should be worrying about. (If you took Ibuprofen in your early pregnancy, please don't start obsessing that your baby could be born without a fully formed head!)

Now I teach that we can replace fear with *trust*. What do you trust? Whom do you trust? Do you trust your body? Your partner, your care provider, your team? Do you trust God? Birth? The process? Start thinking about this. Discovering what you trust *no matter what* will be a giant part of how you stay grounded, whatever happens when your baby comes.

Do you trust your baby? Like, really. Can you truly trust that your baby has a wisdom that is deeper and wider than you can understand and they know what is best for their own birth? For their own life? Can you step outside of your fear and feel a trust that your baby is safe and your baby has a purpose for this lifetime that you cannot change, no matter how much you worry or how much you plan? My hope is you can really sink in and develop a strong connection with your baby, and as you hone your listening skills, you will hear from your baby that they will be born in just the way they need. Even when things feel scary, you can pause, take a breath, and check in with your baby.

What does your baby need in this moment? Is it just a breath? Is it a hug from a support person? Do you need to talk or need to be alone? Is baby hungry or tired? Is something really wrong or are you getting carried away by fear? Again, even as you read, let's check in with baby every time you start to feel fear around labor and birthing.

Place your hand on your baby, take a breath and check in. Notice your own fear, and then ask, is your baby afraid? In most cases, you will sense they are not, they are peaceful and content. They have not learned from external sources to be afraid in the same way you have.

Tap into your baby's energy. Your baby is safe. You are safe. Breathe.

***

WOMB CONNECTION
WHAT DOES YOUR BABY NEED NOW?

*   Next time you are hungry, go to the kitchen and ask your baby what they want to eat. Try not to let your mind answer. Just let your baby's answer come to you.

*   Next time you feel resistance to exercise, ask your baby if there would be a better time or a different type of exercise your baby would prefer.

*   Next time you feel tired, ask your baby what they need. A nap? To go to bed earlier? A few minutes of quiet?

*   Start noticing a few times a day if you can hear what your baby needs in this moment. This requires slowing down and being still, taking a breath, and finding a pause before you do things. It's a new habit and one that will serve you well. You've got this.

www.Genevamontano.com/WisdomFromTheWomb

***

That leaves *pain*. We can replace tension with relaxation and replace fear with trust. What can we replace pain with?

Well, for some people, an epidural is a good option. The epidurals given in many hospitals now can be a helpful tool that allows you to rest and still have movement when it comes time to push. However, an epidural comes with its own set of risks. There is not an easy button for labor. (Remember the old Staples commercials with the easy button? Or am I just aging myself?)

Maybe there is also the possibility that we don't want to replace the pain. The pain we feel during birth can actually act as a guide through the process and help us connect more deeply with our babies. If we can really tune into what our bodies and our babies are feeling during the birth, they will guide us into exactly what we need to do, in many cases. Maybe you'll feel tired, and that means you should rest. Maybe you'll feel best on your hands and knees with pressure on your lower back, and those things are helping to rotate the baby into the perfect position. Your body knows how to give birth, and your baby knows the best way to be born.

For most people, no matter how your birth happens, there will be some pain involved. The great thing about this pain that no one ever tells us is: the pain of childbirth is totally different than any other kind of pain you have experienced throughout your life. In fact, the parts of your brain that are being lit up by the pain of labor are not the same parts that get lit up for other types of pain.

Think about it. The last time you stubbed your toe and were hopping around, cursing and holding your foot and feeling the rising heat of the injury through your body—what is the message your body was trying to give you? It's a warning sign. It's your body telling you something is wrong.

During a normal birth, that is not the case. Everything is working exactly as designed. Your body and your baby are dancing in union, figuring out the steps together. The uterine muscle is contracting, the cervix is opening, the baby is moving down.

Don't get me wrong—Birth feels intense. Perhaps the most intense thing you'll ever experience. If you have been watching YouTube videos where the baby falls out with virtually no effort, a breeze through the air, easy smiles, and inspiring background music... well, you might be disappointed that your birth doesn't look like that. Birth is really freaking hard. But is it "pain"? I guess ultimately that is for each person to decide and determine for themselves during their process.

However, just because we might choose not to replace pain doesn't mean we can't do something about it. Let's think about pain and discomfort in general. When do we feel pain the most and what makes it worse?

Generally, we can tolerate pain more easily if we are well-rested, if we feel loved, if we are not hungry, and don't have other things going on in our bodies that make it more difficult to cope. If I feel sad or angry, when I stub my toe, it hurts a lot! I feel almost personally offended that on top of everything else going on now my toe also has to hurt! That bed frame probably jumped in front of me on purpose, just to spite me. When I feel happy and complete and then stub my toe, it's not as big of a deal.

What things in your life do you notice make pain worse? If you are sick with a cold or the flu, what things make you feel better or worse? Start to take notice of outside factors and how they influence your reaction to discomfort. How does connecting with your baby change your reaction to pain?

Our environment also plays a big role in how we feel about many situations in life. Imagine you are driving in your car with the windows down and your favorite song is playing on the radio. You are enjoying the drive with one of your favorite people next to you. Imagine someone cuts you off in traffic in that scenario. How long does it take you to get over it? How personally do you take it? Now imagine you are driving in your car in stop-and-go traffic, and you forgot your phone, so you can only play the radio, but every station has a commercial on it, and you are late to an appointment. When someone cuts you off in this scenario, how do you react differently than in the previous scenario?

This is an oversimplified analogy, but it still works for birth. Think about your birthing environment. What things will make you feel more relaxed and trusting of yourself, your baby, and the process, and what things will detract from the experience? In the animal kingdom, when a birthing mammal gets scared, her labor will either slow down or stop until she feels safe again. There are protections coded into our DNA to keep our babies safe. If there is a mountain lion nearby, it is not safe to birth a baby. Your body will hold your baby in as long as it is receiving stress hormones.

So, what are the figurative mountain lions in your world? What things cause a reaction of stress or fear when you think about them or are confronted with them? For some women, thinking about a car ride or walking through hospital doors might cause a stress response. Some birthing people might realize that inviting a particular person such as their mother or their sister-in-law, or even the doctor they are seeing, into their birthing space might not be as good an idea as they originally thought. Our environments make a big difference as to how we feel during our birthing process.

In the physical realm, there are also things we can do to mitigate pain. The gate-control theory says that pain travels on different nerve pathways from other sensations. The other sensations, like heat, cold, pressure, pleasure, etc., travel on thicker nerve pathways than pain sensations do. So, these other sensations can actually get to the brain faster than pain and can act as a gate, to keep receptors in the brain from receiving all of the pain messages.

Think about a time when you have burned your finger, remember how you put your finger underneath the cold water and the cold took away the pain. This shows how the sensation of cold travels to the brain first and blocks the sensation of pain. However, the receptors in the brain only accept so many of one particular message before they start letting more pain messages in. So, after you have left your finger in the cold water for a period of time, the sensation of cold is no longer absorbed by the receptors, and the gate is opened for pain messages to come through.

Can you see how this would work during the birthing process as well? Maybe you will find something that is working really well for you—a position that feels comfortable, or your partner touches you in a way that makes you forget you are in labor. After a period of time though, even the things that feel wonderful seem to stop working. It's not usually that the contractions have completely changed or you are no longer able to cope with them in the same way. Often, it is simply that your brain is all filled up with that particular message and is letting more pain messages come in. So, it's time to try something different! Any time a birthing person is struggling or asks for pain relief, before jumping to extremes, I first assume what she is really saying is, "This is not working for me, try something else!"

When we think about labor support and comfort measures, it is often useful to think about stimulating all five senses, to keep the brain distracted. This should not be something the laboring person has to think about, but something that is set up ahead of time that the partner or doula will smoothly incorporate into the birthing process. Some people might find it helpful to make a list of things they like based on each different sense.

**

Sight: what things might be helpful to you that stimulate your sense of sight? Are there pictures of your ancestors or your other children or ultrasound pictures or a color or a place that feel particularly calming or empowering to you? Can you visualize your body opening around your baby's head or your baby being born into your arms?

The sense of sight can be your actual physical sight or it can be in your mind's eye. What can you look at or imagine that you bring into your birthing time that feels magical? When might the lights be dim, and when might you want sunshine in your space? How is baby experiencing birth visually—can you tune into this?

Sound: Do you want music? What kind of music do you think will be most useful for you during your birthing process, if you are feeling tired? What if it's taking longer than you anticipated? Are there certain mantras or affirmations you would like to repeat? Do you want to pray during labor? Can you sing your baby out? What about silence?

Your baby hears the drumbeat of your heart and the tides of your circulation—can these sounds influence the rhythm of your birthing time?

Smell: We don't tend to remember how powerful the sense of smell is. It is actually our only sense that is directly connected to our brain. A scent is the most powerful way to be brought into emotion or a memory. What scents will help you remember your power?

What did your grandma smell like? What makes you feel loved when you smell it? How can you bring those scents into your space? Are there any scents that remind you of a time when you did not feel powerful? Anything that makes you feel nauseous? Laboring people can be very sensitive to smells, so it is important to think about having scents available, but also ensure whatever you are using to provide that smell can be easily disposed of or taken away quickly, if it starts to bother you.

The smell of a newborn baby is intoxicating—it's the smell of another universe, another realm where they came from; it's the scent of your own creative spaces—your womb.

Taste: Contrary to popular belief, it is very important to eat during labor. Your body can burn up to a thousand calories an hour while you are in labor, even if you are just lying in bed. You have to provide energy to your body during this time.

What do you like to eat when you are sick? What things can you swallow easily, without chewing a lot, if that feels like too much during labor? Are there foods your baby has really enjoyed during pregnancy? Nothing is off limits. If you can eat sushi, do it! You can have caffeine, and many midwives even think it's fine to have alcohol. Your baby is fully formed and these things should not affect baby, if you consume them during labor (in moderation and after talking to your care provider, of course).

Some women do not like sweet things while they're in labor, so it might be a good idea to have a variety of options. Some salty things, some savory things, some sweet things. Some solid and some liquid. Some things high in protein to give you sustained energy, and some high in carbs to boost your energy quickly. What does baby want?

Touch: Touch includes just about every other comfort measure you can think of. It includes being touched by another person, as well as the movement of your own body. Most of the time, we have no idea what will feel best in our bodies until we are in the throes of the birthing process. Many women think they will really enjoy massage, and then, once they're in labor, they do not want to be touched. Something like a hip squeeze that doesn't feel very good during pregnancy might feel amazing during early labor and terrible during pushing. We don't know until labor begins. And it will change throughout labor depending on the position of the baby and your own energy levels.

Some people still like to practice a lot of different positioning and massage techniques during pregnancy, and some people don't feel like it's the best use of their time or energy. I believe completely that the baby will tell the birthing person what positions she needs to be in during the birth. A midwife or doula can suggest things that might be helpful, things they see, but they almost never need to be practiced ahead of time.

In all honesty, I feel like this is another myth currently circulated about birth—that you have to do some special combination of different positions in order for your baby to successfully be born and, if you end up with a surprise cesarean birth, it's probably because you didn't do enough positions or maybe didn't try the right one.

Positioning is a tool to use during labor, just like everything else. It is a tool we might pull out of the toolbox or we might leave it in. In my experience, if we just follow the birthing person around, they will probably find all the right positions their baby needs.

The sense of touch also includes *breathing*. Your breath will be your most powerful tool, no matter what type of birth you have. Breath is the only tool you always have access to. Breath will connect you into your womb and remind you of your connection with your baby. Breath brings you into the present moment and grounds you. Practice deep belly breathing, or 3D breathing, which is expanding into all six directions of your ribs as your baby grows, as well as a few other breathing techniques.

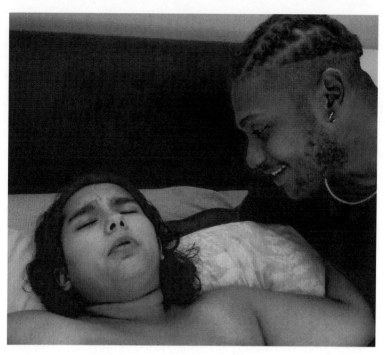

Breaking the Fear-Tension-Pain cycle is one of the most positive things we can do for birthing people. If we can change the narrative around birth to exclude fear and pain, the cycles and patterns that have perpetuated and created harm could be broken. Birthing people could then make choices and have an experience that stems from a place of trust and calm.

Spend some time with your baby about this. When you feel anxious or tense, what things can you do to relax? How can you lessen your perception of pain during birth? Start practicing your tools now. Every time you feel uncomfortable, try one of your distraction tools as well as a deep, grounding breath, to connect to baby. And finally, start exploring your fears so you can lean into trust.

***

Womb Connection
Breath of Light

* Find a comfortable seated position where you can feel your sitz bones evenly on the earth, your spine strong and your heart open. Place one hand on your heart and one hand on your womb.

* We will take one long, deep inhale broken into seven parts through the nose. With each sip, you can envision each of your chakras lighting up, starting at the root chakra and lighting your body up like a rainbow up to your crown chakra.

* Hold the breath gently just for a brief moment at the crown and imagine your third eye like a lighthouse filling your aura, your protective bubble with light. Then exhale slowly out your mouth or your nose. Repeat this breath for seven cycles. When all seven are complete, check in with baby and just notice. Notice how you feel in your body. In your spirit. Notice baby. Does anything feel different?

Cosmic Breath 3

* Find a comfortable seated position where you can feel your sitz bones evenly on the earth, your spine strong, and your heart open. Place one hand on your heart and one hand on your womb.

* Inhale through your nose, exhale through your mouth.

* Inhale through your mouth, exhale through your nose.

* Continue with this pattern for two to three minutes, keeping the length of your inhales and exhales even.

* When you finish, notice how your baby, body, mind, and spirit feel.

This breath balances carbon dioxide and helps us feel more oxygenated. If you were not pregnant, you could hold your breath easily for one minute after completing two minutes of this breath pattern. It is a wonderful pattern to use during labor, especially if you need a distraction.

www.Genevamontano.com/WisdomFromTheWomb

***

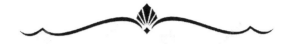

Womb Wisdom: Dace's Story

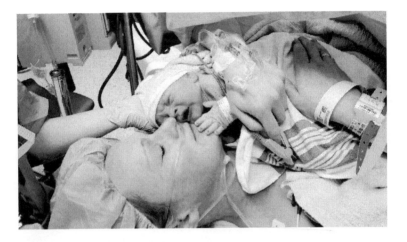

Dace is from Latvia, and we connected when she was pregnant with her second baby. Her first birth had been in the hospital. She'd been convinced by her OB that she was high-risk and needed to be induced at 41 weeks. She felt traumatized by her first birth experience and really wanted to have something different this time. She wanted to feel heard and feel like she was in control of her experience.

She and her partner Dane have one of the best partnerships I've ever seen. You can see how much he adores her and supports her. Even though they are in their late-thirties or early forties, they sit next to each other and have inside jokes and giggle like newly in love teenagers. I love being around them. They also adopted a daughter from Latvia several years ago, and both of the kids were ecstatic to have a new baby in the family.

Dace joked throughout her pregnancy that she was looking for something to be worried about. For a while, it was that her baby was breech. I reassured her time and time again that her baby was head-down. Then for a while she decided to worry about her blood pressure, which was always fine. She was a healthy, strong mother.

As her due date approached, she started getting worried that her baby was not going to come out on time, and she would have to be induced again. I reassured her over and over again that her baby was in control and she was safe. No matter what happened, I would be with her to support her, and she would not have the same experience in the hospital as she'd had the first time.

Anytime I asked how she wanted her birth to look, she said she didn't care. She didn't want to have any expectations so she wouldn't feel disappointed, no matter what happened. The only thing she really wanted was a home birth. As long as the birth happened at home, she would be happy.

Oh, and Christmas lights. She also needed Christmas lights.

Throughout her pregnancy she had a vision of her son being born in the darkness. She pictured him as a Capricorn. Solid and grounded. As her due date passed, she started to have a new vision of him being born in the light. Bright, cold, and airy, like an Aquarius.

I got a call in the middle of the night from Dane. Dace was in labor and things were progressing quickly, so he wanted me to come over. I called my team, and we all went over to their house.

We got the pool set up while Dace labored on the toilet.

She said she felt like a goddess as she floated in the birthing pool with Dane nearby and her team of midwives lounging in the next room, ready to support her every need.

When she asked me to check her, I found she was about 5 to 6 cm, and there was a bulging bag of water. The head felt a little funny, like I could feel very pronounced suture lines. I was thinking maybe it was going to be a really tight squeeze for baby to make it out. I told the family that the head felt different than I was expecting, but that everything seemed fine and she could continue laboring at home.

After a few more hours, Dace asked me to check her again, and while I was checking, her water broke. This time when I felt the head without the cushion of water, I realized the reason the head felt so funny was because it was a butt. I was feeling the sacrum and a little bit of the baby's butt crack. We made the move over to a friendly hospital so she could possibly deliver her breech baby vaginally.

Once we got settled at the hospital, Dace's contractions almost completely stopped. I checked in with her about what was going on, and she told me her mother had delivered Dace breech vaginally, and she had been told her entire life how she had almost broken her mother's body. How her mother had never fully recovered from delivering a breech baby.

I asked Dace if she felt like she could connect with her mom during this time. I thought maybe the baby was breech so she could connect with her mom's experience. Dace's mom had passed away that year, while Dace was pregnant. After I suggested this, many tears followed.

Dace was not sure if she was safe or if her baby was safe. She was unsure how to proceed—whether to try to get labor going again and have a vaginal birth or just have a cesarean.

I got Dace set up in the bathtub after some deep heart-to-heart conversations and asked her if it was okay if I left for a few hours. I needed to get my car, which I had left at their house in order to ride with them to the hospital. Dace was not having contractions, and she felt comfortable with me leaving while she decided how she wanted to proceed with her birth.

A few hours later, I got a call from Dane that they had decided to go ahead with a cesarean. I was feeling terrible. The one thing Dace didn't want was to go to the hospital, and instead of having the beautiful, healing home birth she wanted, she ended up with a cesarean in the hospital.

My insides were wrecked, thinking they must be so angry with me and disappointed in my skills, since I didn't know their baby was breech throughout pregnancy. Even when she was worried and asked me about her baby's position, I had falsely reassured her that everything was perfect! These are the moments where I beat myself up—I question every decision I've ever made about being a midwife. I was exhausted from sleeping only three hours in a forty-hour period. From this state, I was imagining all the worst, knowing their exhaustion was greater than my own.

When I arrived at the hospital after the cesarean, I found the happiest, shiniest Dace and Dane I could imagine. They were so in love with their new baby and so happy with their experience. When I started to apologize that I had missed the breech position, Dace told me I didn't miss it. It was hidden from me. She said, if I had told her that her baby was breech, she would have worried through the entire pregnancy instead of enjoying it. She never would have had her goddess experience at home.

She felt healed from her previous birth and connected to

her mother. Dane had realized that Dace's vision of little Ziggy being born into cold, bright light was a vision of the operating room. Ziggy had told them ahead of time how he would be born.

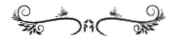

FACING FEAR

SOMETHING ABOUT BABIES makes us want to take care of them. It is hardwired into mammals to care for their young until they can care for themselves. We usually only see one side of this story: how great it is that parents care for their babies. But what about the babies? How does the baby *feel*, knowing it has to rely on this larger version of itself to meet its needs? Are they ever afraid?

It seems newborns sit squarely in trust. I can't really think of anything that seems to frighten them. Dogs bark around them, people yell, doors slam; they ride in moving vehicles at 75 mph, they are carted around in plastic carriers with their heads flailing all over the place, and nothing phases them. Spiders, clowns, heights—no problem. In fact, not only are they not afraid, they often make the big people around them feel more brave and peaceful.

Babies do, however, have certain instincts they are born with that are designed to keep them safe. The instinct to breathe is number one. Eating is a close second. The instinct to stay alive is strong, and only when they feel their ability to live is threatened do we see newborns react. From the moment they are born, they are programmed to survive.

Besides breathing and eating, they also like to be close

to someone big—another survival instinct. Somewhere in their newborn mammalian brains, they know, if they are left alone with no one else around, there is a chance they could become another mammal's prey. But they are not "afraid" this will happen; they aren't lying in their mother's arms, fretting about a lion coming to eat them. They just follow an instinct when they realize they have been put down and are vulnerable to the greater world.

They cry when they are alone, so a big person will come be close to them and keep them protected. They cry when they are hungry, so someone will give them sustenance to keep them alive, but they do not seem afraid the next meal isn't coming. Newborns are the epitome of peace and trust. Babies have an innate need to feel safe. But they fully trust their every need will be provided for, until they have an experience that teaches them otherwise.

When we observe toddlers, we see they believe they are safe until an adult tells them they are not. They play, they frolic, enjoying the ecstasy that exploring their body and their world brings them. Then, in their uncoordinated toddler-ness, sometimes they fall. In that initial moment of surprise that they've lost control of the body, they make a brief assessment of themselves, see if they are safe, see if the body still responds to their will, and then get back to enjoying. That is, unless an adult intervenes.

When an adult rushes over in the hurried way adults do, worried about the toddler's safety, full of anxiety and fear that certainly something has happened to damage the body, the toddler starts to wonder if maybe they aren't safe after all. There must be something wrong, if the adult, whom the toddler trusts, is so panicked! A fear of falling begins to develop, because the fall has triggered a response in the adult, even if the toddler at first thought he was okay when he checked in with himself.

From now on, this toddler is more likely to cry and express both fear and pain after a fall. This toddler has been taught to be afraid of a fall. The brain has learned a response of fear, in order to keep the toddler safe, whether or not frolicking with joy is actually something to be afraid of.

You were also born with an innate need to feel safe. In fact, your body cannot work in all the beautiful and brilliant ways it was designed, cannot heal itself or function at its best, when it does not feel safe. Fear is an instinct that helps keep us safe. However, many of our fears are not founded in truth or even in personal experience. Somewhere along the way, the instincts built into your mammalian brain to keep you safe might have been triggered in a way that created fears of not being safe, even when the situation at hand might not have actually been dangerous.

Most people have been taught, on a subconscious level through personal or shared experiences, what things they should be afraid of. Your brain has learned a response and wants to keep you safe. Fears are not something you were born with; you *learned* to be afraid. Your parents and your teachers and the media taught you specific things you should or should not fear.

If this is a new concept for you, it might be helpful to spend some time exploring this idea. Why are you actually afraid of a certain thing? Who else do you know who shares that fear and when and where was that fear developed? Now that you are an adult, you get to weed through the things that could truly be dangerous and the things you have been conditioned to fear.

Giving birth is high on the list of fears for many pregnant

or fertile people. This is a fear that has most likely been taught, either by cultural norms, the media, or by your family. Your body was perfectly designed to give birth, just as it was perfectly designed to breathe and eat and frolic with joy. Fear around your body's perfect design to give birth is not innate, but it is valid and needs to be addressed, in order to move past it.

Warning: many subjects in this chapter could be triggering. Fear has a way of doing that. Remember, your brain is just trying to keep you safe.

We live in a unique time in regards to birth. We have the lowest mortality rates that have ever existed, and yet we also have the most fear around childbirth.

When we talk about birth, we have to address fear first, because your number-one instinct as a pregnant person is to be safe and keep your baby safe. There are myriad things, both real and imagined, that may make you feel unsafe. I would like to address some of these things, knowing I cannot possibly guess every fear every person has.

My hope is, while some of these might be triggering, you will sit with each one and determine for yourself, while checking in with your baby and trying to feel the same peace and trust they feel, which are fears you have been taught, and which are instincts that are in place to keep you safe. As fears come up for you, I hope you will sit with them, explore them, and honor them, so you can move past them. When it feels intense, check in with your baby. How does your baby feel about this fear? Are they trying to communicate with you that there may be a legitimate reason to be concerned or afraid? Or has your brain gone on a little fear trip?

One of the most common reasons people are afraid of childbirth is because it is unknown. Most people in the 21st

century have never attended a birth prior to anticipating their own. We live in little isolated boxes, and we do not usually get the opportunity to even hear the true stories of other people's births. We hear the horror stories, and we see the births on TV, which must fit into a time slot between commercial breaks and are written to provide tension, drama, action, or sometimes even comedy. We have lost touch with what it is to be a pregnant or birthing person surrounded by community. We have no idea what to expect during pregnancy and especially during birth.

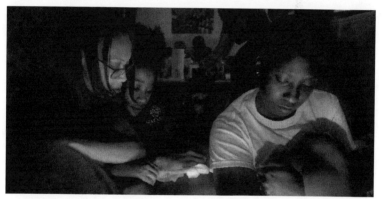

Until recent history, a young pregnant woman would commune with her pregnant family and neighbors in close confines. She would have a real sense of the discomforts and worries of pregnancy. Eventually, she would hear the moans of her neighbor during birth, bring her food postpartum, watch her breastfeed her newborn. She would know closely what childbirth looks like, sounds like, smells like.

A video of an animated uterus cannot teach a pregnant person what birth will be like any more than a picture of a vulva and a penis can teach her what sex will be like. Some things you can only truly know through lived experience. Sharing experiences with community members you know and trust is a close second. Witnessing a birth does not mean you know how it will feel when you are in it, but it does help take the fear away by normalizing it.

It is taboo to even talk about these things in our culture. Many birthing people don't even share with their closest friends or relatives what happens inside the delivery room. I am forty-two years old, have been a birth worker for over fifteen years, talk about birth with everyone I encounter night and day, and only found out last week that I was delivered by forceps. I'm not kidding. My mom just told me *last week*!

People generally do not share their intimate birth experiences in our culture. Sure, you can go on YouTube and see births—but you can't ask these people how it felt or what they were afraid of and how that fear resolved. Many birth videos leave us with more question than answers. More fear than peace. Can I do it? What if I can't do it? What if I'm not strong enough? What if I'm not as graceful as these women? What if I'm too loud? What if something bad happens?

Let's walk through a little bit of birth history to see how we got to this place where people are afraid of birth. Until the early 20th century, women were mostly left to their own devices and trusted to handle birth in whatever way they had been handling it since the origin of our species. Throughout time, women have been attended by other women—by some version of midwives. It is said that midwifery is the second oldest profession, prostitution being the first. Those midwives might have been medicine women, highly trained and revered healers. Or they might have been mothers and aunts who had birthed many babies themselves and were now assisting the process.

In the era of Hippocrates in ancient Greece, Western

medicine became a field of study. At that time, and for hundreds of years after, Western medicine started spreading throughout the world. However, women were still in charge of their own health and, therefore, pregnancy and birth, because the study of Western medicine mainly dealt with men's health. It was actually viewed with disdain for a doctor to consider treating a woman, especially in the nether regions.

Most doctors considered it beneath them to attend the average birth, because it was not a medical event. Babies were conceived without much assistance, other than maybe prayer or a little bit of plant medicine. They grew in the womb without assistance, and they came out of the woman's body without assistance. What is medical in that scenario? Things that happen as normal bodily functions did not generally gain the attention of a medical doctor.

(Have you ever thought about having a doctor come assist you take a poop? Or do you usually think your body has that handled, even when it takes a little longer than expected? There could come an extreme time when you decide you need medical intervention for your poop. In that case, a doctor is a great choice. Until then, you might try being patient, maybe eating different foods, hydrating, or even an enema—all things you can handle on your own. Birth is also a natural bodily function, which in the past was not seen as a medical event that required a doctor. But I digress.)

Around 1200 years ago, as medicine became more highly regarded and indoctrinated religion became more and more important in Western culture and the colonized world, midwives started to be regarded as witches. They understood plant medicine and spirit medicine and were considered to be practicing outside of religious norms. Because of this, they were persecuted, and almost all midwives and traditional healers throughout Europe were killed. The medical doctors needed people to practice their new trade on. So, if you were discovered seeking the services of these "witches," you could be found guilty by association and also face death. This is not something readily taught in history classes, but this is what happened during the Inquisition. Many thousands of women were killed, their wisdom and skills put to rest with them. (Remember, history is taught by the oppressors.)

In America, many of the women killed in the Salem witch trials were midwives. Natural birth started to be seen as a belief in witchcraft. It's hard to believe something that has happened since the beginning of human existence could be seen as worthy of punishment.

This did not happen by accident. People in power who wanted money decided to make midwifery something to be feared, so they could have control over the bodies, minds, and money of their subjects. But public perception is such that, if the midwives are murdered, they must have done something wrong. It can then be inferred that natural birth and natural medicine are wrong and should be feared. Fear is the most efficient way to control people. We keep people "safe" by creating fear around the things we want them to stay away from. *Witches, Midwives, and Nurses* by Barbara Ehrenreich is a rich resource to learn more about this phenomenon.

If you are afraid of natural birth, at least some of this was taught to you by powerful white men who want your money. As mentioned, in early 20th century America, almost everyone was born at home. Many white midwives had been killed and the rest pushed underground, but someone still had to catch the babies, so most of the midwives who were attending births were either indigenous midwives who were here when the colonizers arrived or they were Grand midwives, black slaves who had retained the wisdom from their native lands or had it passed down to them from their predecessors, other slave women. We owe everything we still know about natural birth and midwifery to these women!

At that point in time, the American Medical Association was not very highly regarded. The schools in America were lacking, and most doctors who trained in America had to go back to Europe to get further education, if they wanted to be seen as legitimate. Since birth was seen as women's work, it was not really part of the education a doctor received at that point. Somewhere along the way, someone realized that if more women birthed in the hospital, the doctors could learn obstetrics. They also realized how many babies are born and what a missed opportunity this was for money making!

Nowadays, birth accounts for twenty-five percent of hospital admittances. If a hospital can gain your loyalty during your birthing time, you are more likely to go back to that hospital for other care your family needs. Even when they are treated poorly, many people return to the same place they had their baby, because it is what they know, and humans find comfort in what is familiar to them. Hospitals started to figure out it was a cash cow to care for pregnant and birthing people.

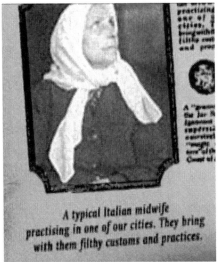

A typical Italian midwife practising in one of our cities. They bring with them filthy customs and practices.

Thus began a smear campaign against midwives in the United States. Around the big cities, there were flyers hung that depicted a poor, immigrant, dirty, black, or indigenous midwife on one side and a clean-cut, white-coat, short-haired male on the other side. The flyers reported that the midwives brought with them filth and dirty traditions and customs. Traditional midwives had also always helped women with plant medicine for unwanted pregnancies and birth control—yet another reason the Puritans who were colonizing America demonized midwives.

Within a few years, anyone who had enough money started to move to the hospital to give birth. Anyone who had privilege or was white did whatever they could to show their worth by birthing in a hospital and not with a "dirty" midwife. (Interestingly enough, we now have the opposite problem in the US. Out-of-hospital birth is generally not covered by insurance, so now, it is typically only the privileged who can afford to or are offered the opportunity to have a birth at home or in a birth center.)

To be fair, the rate of death has gone down since the majority of births moved to the hospital. In 1900, the infant mortality rate was about ten percent. Today, it is less than one percent, no matter where you choose to birth. Overall, you are giving birth in a relatively safe time. What a blessing for you! You can feel some relief that you are far safer giving birth now than you could be at any other time in recorded history.

If your baby needs to be born in the hospital, there is now more awareness of patient rights, informed choice, and doulas who can help you advocate for yourself and ask questions about your care. If you choose to have your baby out of hospital, the ability to get to a hospital quickly in an emergency definitely lowers the risk of death for both moms and babies.

Side note: the statistics for women who are not white are far worse than those for women and babies who are white. If you are not white, you do have more reason to be afraid of birth. In America, your chances of dying or having your baby die in childbirth are at least three times higher.[2] This makes it even more important for you to be somewhere where you feel safe, where you are listened to and respected. You are the expert on your own body, and you have a connection with your baby that no one else has.

When Serena Williams had complications during birth and postpartum, no one believed her. And she is rich and powerful! The average woman of color in America has a hard time making sure she is treated fairly and listened to. Women of color: Please know that you matter, and you have the right to have your voice heard. Keep talking until you find someone who will listen. We can't lose another infant or mother of color because they were silenced by a care provider who didn't listen.

**

Here are some of the great birthing ideas that were invented by men: It is speculated that, in France in the 1600s, King Louis XIV was the trendsetter who came up with the

brilliant idea that women should birth lying down. King
Louis XIV was a very sexual human, it seems. In addition to
his many wives, he also had babies with many of his servants
and perhaps a few commoners.

It seems the king was not only interested in making
babies, he also had a fascination with seeing them be born.
At that time in Europe, women traditionally gave birth on a
birthing stool, and they wore long skirts so as to remain
modest and adhere to the cultural and religious norms of the
time. (Honestly, probably also super uncomfortable.) In this
position, Louis could not spectate sufficiently! So, he
required his offspring to be born of a woman lying flat on
her back on a pedestal, with her legs up in the air. As the
other nobility and then the commoners heard about this,
they figured if this was the best practice for the king's
children, it was probably how they should do it, as well.

Before this, very few
women would ever have
chosen to give birth lying
on their backs with their
feet up in the air. It goes
against gravity, as well as
the body's innate sense. In
normal birth, the sacrum
will lift up to allow the baby
to have more room during
the fetal ejection reflex at
the end of the pushing
phase, but if you're lying on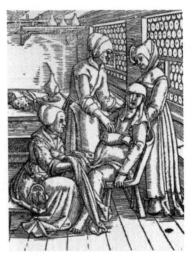
your back, it is not possible for the sacrum to lift.

There is nothing about you being on your back that
makes birth easier, in most cases. It does make it easier for

doctors to do episiotomies and use forceps. As those things gained popularity, so did the lithotomy position. The person delivering your baby may have learned that birth should happen this way from the attending physician during their training, who learned it from another doctor, who learned it from Louis XIV's doctor. They might be unwilling or maybe just haven't had the chance to learn a different way. You could be the person who gives another doctor their first opportunity to catch a baby in a different position. Change is created through consumer demand, one birth, one baby, one doctor at a time. How does your baby want to be born?

The father of modern gynecology, J Marion Sims, is credited with inventing the speculum, as well as perfecting various vaginal surgeries. Before this, it was not considered necessary to visually inspect a woman's vagina for health. His research was conducted on Black slave women, without their consent and without anesthesia. Most everything we know about how your vagina and your pelvis "should look," how big or small they "should be," was invented by a man who took advantage of slave women, a man engaging in medical rape. Yes. Be enraged.

It used to be standard practice to do prenatal X-rays on women, to see if it looked like the pelvis was adequate to birth their baby. Turns out, X-rays can be harmful to fetal cells. It also turns out you can't measure how much the pelvic cavity will stretch or open during the birthing process. The female body actually opens around the baby to allow birth to happen. Maybe your body is just perfect and we don't even need to know what it looks like internally or how it measures—your baby will still be born without a problem! But because the female body was (or is?) a mystery to male doctors, they needed to invent ways to make it understandable. Ways that do not work.

If you are afraid of the way birth and women's health care are right now, it's for good reason. You were never meant to be cared for in some of these ways. The medical field is still researching and experimenting to find the best way for your baby to be born. Most recently, they have decided that 39 weeks is the ideal time for a baby to be born, and many doctors are recommending labor be started artificially at that time, regardless of how well the pregnant person and baby are doing.[3] Is it possible that you and your baby already know how to have the best birth without anyone intervening? If you and your baby are connected, your birth will be perfect—perfect for what you and your baby need.

In the 1950s, there was a hospital that made a cute black-and-white birth education video for their patients to watch prior to being admitted into the hospital for childbirth. It gave them a virtual tour of labor and delivery, told them what to pack, when to come to the hospital—things of that sort. The narrator of this video tells women not to worry about their care, their doctor will take care of everything, and all they need to bring with them is their make-up, so they can look pretty. (I am not making this up: you can see this video on YouTube—*Labor and Delivery 1950.*)

In the spring of 2020, I saw a billboard advertising one of the biggest health networks in the major city where I live, that says, "Choosing your baby's first outfit is hard. Choosing who delivers her shouldn't be." Basically, you don't need to think about anything or know about anything, just make sure your baby looks cute when you leave. This infuriates me. Twenty-first-century pregnant people are intelligent and have access to more information than ever before. They can make choices that matter a lot more than what their baby is wearing.

Now, as you may remember, I am a strong believer that you cannot know enough to have a perfect birth. But you can certainly know enough to make a wise decision about who delivers your baby. (By the way, your baby does not need to be delivered. You, as the birthing person, birth your baby. Someone catches your baby. UPS delivers the cute outfit. The definition of the word "deliver," during the time it was first used in reference to childbirth, is "to save, rescue, or set someone or something free." Basically saying, the doctor is saving your baby from your body. So, the same body that built, protected, and nurtured this baby for nine months is now somehow dangerous, and your baby needs to be saved from it? I don't think so.)

You *are* the most powerful and wise person in this birthing experience. You are the *only* one who can know, with the guidance of your baby, what this experience needs to look like. You have a lot more to do than just pick your baby's outfit. Your baby could not care less what outfit they wear. This is your baby's birth—and it matters.

These are just a few examples of how a misunderstanding of the female body has led to the learned fear many pregnant people have that they will be unable to handle birth. The field of obstetric medicine has studied the female body as "other," meaning, it has primarily been studied in relation to how it is different from the male body, which has been considered the standard, or the norm. The female body has been measured and calculated in terms of how everything "should" work.

But this is not the way the feminine flows. The feminine

prefers things happen in their own time and in their own way, with gentle acceptance. If it is hard for you to wrap your head around birth, it could be because birth cannot be distilled into a book or a class or a graph or a thirty-minute appointment. The reason you can't find answers to the questions that keep you up at night with anxiety and fear is because no book has the answer for you. The only way to work through that fear is to go through it. See your fear, acknowledge it, shine light on it, love it, walk next to it. This is the feminine way. Return to your baby: is your baby afraid? Can you sit in the trust that the answers you seek, the peace you seek, are already within you? The wisdom is in your womb.

***

Here are some other things I hear people are afraid of: What if the cord is around the neck? Isn't that a medical emergency? Rarely it is. In most cases, about twenty-five to thirty percent of births, having a cord around the neck is not a big deal. That's right: twenty-five to thirty percent of babies are born with a cord around their neck, and it is non-eventful. The baby either just slides out and someone untangles it from the baby's body, or if it is tighter and not allowing baby to move down, it is slipped over the baby's head; in extreme cases, the cord can be cut on the perineum, while the baby is coming out. Most people haven't heard stories about healthy babies being born with a cord around their neck, but it happens so many times every day.

What if I poop during labor? If there is fecal matter in your rectum at the time of birth, your baby's head will push it out. It usually comes out in pellets, like rabbit poop, not like a big, giant turd. Some women have gotten enemas or refrained from eating during labor to keep this from happening.

I don't recommend starving yourself or your baby out of fear of pooping. You'd have to keep food out of your system for quite some time to ensure nothing is in your rectum at the time of birth. Everybody poops! It's one of the things we don't love sharing with others, especially strangers, but I guarantee, whoever might see you poop during labor has also pooped.

Think about your baby. When they are born, they will poop, and you will be so happy to see that their tiny body works perfectly! You will celebrate and investigate poop in a whole new way. Your baby wants you to love your own bodily functions in the same way. Teach them to poop healthily by honoring your own poop. Trust me, it's a better option than keeping all that poop inside.

What if I tear? Vaginal tissue, like penile tissue, is designed to stretch. Ina May Gaskin talks about meditating on how big your vagina can get. Think like a dude: I have the biggest, most powerful vagina this baby has ever seen! (It is true!)

About half of first-time birthers tear. The vaginal tissue is mucous membrane, similar to the tissue inside your mouth. This type of tissue is very sensitive but heals very quickly! Just like when you bite the inside of your cheek—it hurts like heck, but it feels better in a short time. About half of the women you see walking around with their kids have had a tear in their vagina or perineum, and they are perfectly normal. You can't tell in any way that they tore. Their partner usually can't, either. It is important you give your body time to heal after a tear, but trust that your body was designed perfectly for birth, and if it tears, it knows how to heal, given the proper tools—rest, nutrition, hydration, love.

Sometimes, we ourselves are not afraid at all, but our loved ones are, so we feel forced into making decisions we would not otherwise make, in order to appease the people around us. I do find it important that your support people be on board with the decisions you make surrounding your birth. If they don't feel comfortable, it will be very difficult for you to feel comfortable when it comes time to birth the baby.

I also know, if your birth does not go as planned and you did not feel comfortable with the location or the care team you chose, in order to keep everyone else happy, you will question this decision. Probably for the rest of your life. You will never get a chance to go back and do it another way. You will never know if that particular birth could have been different if you had followed your instincts. Even if you choose a different type of experience for your next baby, you will always wonder.

It is worth taking the time to really explore in depth with your friends and family, if you are not feeling safe with the choices you are being faced with. At the end of the day, it's your body and it should be your decision. Is your baby telling you they want to be born a certain way? Are you honoring your baby's wishes?

Stephanie, whom I told you about earlier, her mother-in-law is a doctor, so they chose not to tell her they were planning a home birth. They did not tell her until after the baby was born.

When I went to visit them at four or five days postpartum, Stephanie said she had had a very emotional day the previous day, because her mother-in-law was so angry with her and her husband for making such a, in her opinion, dangerous choice. Stephanie had been crying most of the previous day, because her family was upset with the decision she had made, even though the birth went beautifully and she and her baby were perfectly healthy.

No matter what choices you make, you eventually will have to take ownership of those choices. Long-term, an angry mother-in-law may or may not be easier to deal with than recovering physically and emotionally from a second surgery. It's something each person has to decide for themselves. Stephanie does not regret her choice.

No matter how you birth, you will have to make some hard decisions, and ultimately, you will be responsible for the consequences. This is why it is so important to really spend time listening to your baby and to your intuition. You have an innate wisdom that will put you in the right place at the right time. Your baby shares this wisdom and can communicate their needs to you, if you pause and listen.

If you have had a previous birth that felt traumatic to you in some way, it might be even more difficult to feel safe during this pregnancy. It will take a lot of inner work and connecting with your baby for you to trust that this experience can and will be different. I am willing to make you a promise: this pregnancy and this birth will be different. I don't know how it will be different. But I *guarantee* it will be.

Giving birth to a different baby is similar to having sex with a different partner. When we have sex for the first time, we might have one particular experience and then think we have experienced sex. But perhaps, when we have sex again with a different partner or even with the same partner but under different circumstances, we realize how very different one sexual experience can be from another.

In this pregnancy, you have a different partner, a

completely different human inside of you than you did last time. Even if they have the same parents, their DNA is different. They have their own consciousness and their own plan for this lifetime. Even if you schedule a cesarean on the same date with the same doctor at the same location, I guarantee you this experience is going to be different. As much as you can, try to let go of all expectations for this birth. Try to connect to what this particular baby needs and wants, instead of getting stuck in the lived experience you had with the previous partner!

Bear with me here, we are about to get real. Get down to where the real fear is buried. Nobody wants to talk about it, but there is a small chance someone has a negative outcome or even dies during birth. This is the nitty-gritty of fear. This is the part where your innate instincts come in and tell you there could be danger.

The fear of death is what creates the fear of birth. The fear of death is what creates every other fear around birth (and really, every fear in your life). Take a deep breath and let that sink in. You are afraid of birth on an instinctual level, because you are afraid that you or your baby might die.

We have been taught in our culture to fear death. If we can address the fear of death, we have the possibility to take away the fear of birth (and really all of our fears). Our society is terrified of death. We will do anything to stay alive. No matter the cost monetarily or energetically, we put a high value on not dying.

Above all the guarantees I make in this book, I put the highest bet on this one: no matter what you do, you are going to die. It probably will not be in childbirth. But your brain does know that is a possibility. Sometimes, despite all the amazing technology and very smart, talented doctors and all the prayers and trust and everything else we do, babies or moms still die. Your body knows this. Facing your fear of death will ultimately change every aspect of your life, but especially your fears around birth.

Birth gives us the unique opportunity to face our fear of death. There is a study involving cancer patients who were on their deathbed. Some of them were given mind-altering substances that induced a feeling of losing control of their minds for a short period of time. Those who were given this medicine reported they no longer had a fear of death. They reportedly lived out their final days with a sense of peace and joy they did not previously have.[4]

During birth, we are given the opportunity to lose our minds. To step out of our thinking brains and let the hormones of birth take over. Some people liken the experience of labor to a psychedelic experience, where they feel out of control. In my experience, the people who have been able to let go and lose control have had the least fear and report the most positive birth experiences.

Until recently, it was expected that some babies would not make it. For example, farmers had fifteen children so that when a few of them passed during birth or at a young age, it didn't affect the workload as much. Death has always been a part of birth, and it still is. That being said, I want to reiterate that you live in the safest time we have known to give birth. There are approximately four million babies born on this planet every year. That means at the same time you are birthing, about 250 other babies are born that same minute. Chances are you and your baby are going to be safe! The maternal death rate is around two per 1,000 births worldwide, and the neonatal death rate is about seventeen per 1,000, with a third of those occurring within the first day of life. Most of these are genetic anomalies, when the baby's body was incompatible with life. It's no one's "fault."

I believe each soul chooses to be incarnated, chooses their parents, and chooses the experiences in this lifetime that will help it learn and grow in the particular way it wants. We cannot always understand in our finite human minds why things happen. But I believe, when a baby dies, it knew coming into this life, before it entered the womb, that this was the experience it needed for its own growth and for the highest good of all beings.

I believe, when a mother dies, she has agreed before coming into this body that she would learn and grow from these particular experiences, and the baby also needed the experience that not having a mother would teach. Perhaps it is for ancestral healing or for some higher good on the planet.

These beliefs in no way take away the immense grief associated with a loss. No one knows pain more than a parent who has lost a child or a family who has lost their mother. Anyone who experiences a loss during pregnancy or birth or of a young child will deal with the trauma of that experience and see the world through a different lens for the rest of their lives. It never goes away, though it will fade and change over time. The suffering associated with loss is very real. This suffering is, however, enough on its own. Could it be that the anxiety we cause ourselves fearing the possibility of loss is an unnecessary suffering?

In no way do I want to minimize the fear of death. It is the last thing any of us wants to consider when we are expecting a new life. I have been blessed not to have a firsthand understanding of death in childbirth. So, while I cannot fully understand, I do feel deeply the immense grief that death carries. More deeply than grief, however, I feel a trust and knowing that our souls have a higher purpose. Maybe, if we can learn to lean into that trust and knowing, we will someday be able to understand the "why" more clearly when things happen that we do not expect.

Medicine cannot save you from your birth. In fact, there are likely to be more problems the more that interventions are introduced. Many deaths and injuries result from iatrogenic causes every year. One study reports it as the third highest cause of death in the US.[5] Of course, if there is something out of the ordinary going on, you absolutely want a doctor with tools and medicine nearby! But if you are having a low-risk pregnancy, you have the responsibility to think about your options and where you and your baby will feel safest.

When you are pregnant, you might be bombarded with stories of emergency cesarean births and other stories where someone says they certainly would have died if not for the quick reaction of the medical staff. I am totally grateful that medical staff are able to act as quickly as they can to save people in many cases. However, sometimes we don't get to hear the beginning of the story.

Often, these emergency births begin with something like an induced labor—a baby who wasn't quite ready to come and was being forced out. We know that one of the side effects of Pitocin, the drug used to cause the uterus to contract so that it dilates, is contractions that are not always handled well by the baby. When a woman goes into labor on her own, her body is generally producing the perfect strength of contractions that her baby can handle at that time. When contractions are medically induced, we don't always know what the perfect strength is for this particular baby, and sometimes babies say, "No thank you." Their heartrate drops, and an emergency cesarean becomes necessary.

Or maybe the baby was stuck in the wrong position because the woman was never educated about things she could do during pregnancy to help her baby have the most efficient birth possible. Our 21st-century lifestyle is not nearly as conducive to easy birth as it was prior to the 19th century. The care provider might have to use tools to assist the baby out, but if the baby does not tolerate this, again we end up with an emergency situation.

There are true emergencies in childbirth. About one to two percent of cesarean births are true emergencies. The other emergency cesareans that you hear about are not true emergencies, but unplanned cesarean births. The care team decided that the safest way to proceed with birth would be surgically, and it is often the right decision at that time. However, it is usually not an emergency. This is an important distinction. You can decide if it is in the best interest of you and your baby to have a cesarean birth, or get any other medical intervention you, with the input of your baby, and your care provider determine is best, without it being an emergency. It is of the utmost importance that you have a care team you trust.

In terms of your instinct to be safe, for most women and most babies, a cesarean does not feel safe. In your mammalian brain, there is a knowledge that being sliced open means death. Cesareans were named after Julius Caesar, whose mother died in childbirth after he was saved by being cut out of her belly. Until recently, either mom or baby would generally not survive this type of birth.

If you are faced with a cesarean, whether it is planned,

unplanned, or emergency, your body probably does not feel safe. Even if, on a logical level, you know it is the right thing to do, there will most likely be some level of trauma response. It will take time for your body, mind, spirit, and those of your baby to integrate that no one died. Give yourself and your baby lots of extra time and love, if cesarean birth is part of your story.

Our society is very fond of finding someone to blame whenever anything goes wrong, especially if someone is hurt or dies. Who would you blame if your baby died? Who is responsible for the health and safety of you and your baby? People who are choosing a birth center, home birth, or especially, unassisted birth generally have a lot more conversations with their babies, their partners, and themselves about responsibility.

Ultimately, you are responsible for your own care, no matter where you choose to birth. In order to have an empowered birth, you have to own all aspects of your care. If you are birthing at a hospital, you are responsible for making your voice and your baby's voice heard. You cannot sit quietly and hope for the best outcome. You have to ask questions, demand informed choice, find your power, maybe hire a doula. If you have an unassisted birth, it's pretty difficult to sue yourself if something goes wrong.

Whatever choices you make, I encourage every birthing person, every parent, to sit with the responsibility inherent in birth. Have a real heart-to-heart with your baby. Are they safe? What do they need to have the best birth experience? Are you feeling fear? Why? Is it a learned fear or an instinct designed to keep you safe? What needs to change to let that fear go? Are you comfortable with the choices you have made thus far? Is your baby?

I know this is not a fun topic, but I do believe it is important, because most people are at least a little bit afraid of dying in childbirth, even if they only know it on a subconscious level. There is something innately written in us that knows birth is a big deal, that it matters for ourselves and for our babies, even when it is not life or death.

Non-gestational parents are often more acutely aware of the worry that their partner or their baby might die than the gestational parent is. When I ask a dad what his biggest fear about birth is, the most common answer is that someone will die. The gestational parent does generally have more of an innate sense of trust and knowing the baby is going to be okay and so will they. Most of the moms I ask say their biggest fear is that they won't be able to tolerate the pain. However, that innate trust and knowing of safety doesn't necessarily make the fear go away.

This fear is real, and you, in a sense, will indeed die during childbirth. Just as young men throughout history have been required to endure certain rites of passage to prove their manhood and worthiness to their tribe, so do young women endure pregnancy and childbirth to become warriors in their own right. We may not have to go out and kill wild game or survive three nights alone in the darkness, but we certainly spend many hours in a place where we feel scared and alone and have to face our fears.

Sometimes, the hours turn into days, and no one can tell us for sure when it will end. Even when the birth is very fast, it can be so intense, many women have an almost out-of-body experience, because they feel so out of control when birth happens that fast. There's nothing easy about a fast birth, and most birthing people who experience one definitely at some point wonder if they might die or whether they can possibly survive the wild ride their body is taking them on.

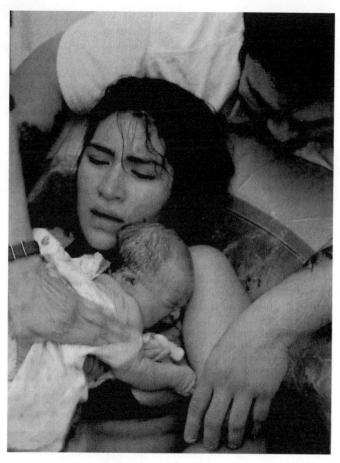

The truth is, no matter what the experience looks like, no one can save you when you are in your birthing time. Your partner, your doula, your doctor, even an epidural cannot take your fear away. They can help remind you that you are safe, but they can't remove the sensations or thoughts you have. It's up to you to decide if you will pause, connect with your baby, determine what is necessary to stay safe and calm as you continue the process, or whether you will succumb to your fears.

You, like all the women before you, will have to face your fears at some point during your pregnancy or birth. Some part of you will die during your birth. Even if this is your tenth baby, you will not come out of this birth unchanged. You can have the easiest birth ever known to mankind and I promise, the experience will change you. Physically, mentally, spiritually, emotionally... You will not be the same person after your baby is born. You will be both stronger and more tender. Wiser and in full knowledge that you know very little. More full of love and somehow also more vulnerable than ever.

Phew. I told you this was going to get real. Take a deep breath. Feel your baby inside you. Feel your heart connected to your baby's heart. Slow down, and really feel that connection.

It is magical to be born. You and your baby will be born as new humans together. You get to experience a whole new life with this new being who is blessing your journey through the wild ride we call birth.

Breathe. You are safe. Trust your baby. Feel the intensity, and let it be there. Let it change you. (This is great practice for birth, when every intense wave will change your body as you open up around your baby, preparing you to die to the old and be born anew.) You were made for this. Your baby is leading the way. You've got this.

***

WOMB CONNECTION
FEAR BALANCING KRIYA

✶ Find a comfortable seat where you can feel your sitz bones connecting to the earth, to the chair, or to the cushion beneath you. Draw energy from the earth up through your root chakra. Feel your pelvis and spine in a neutral position. Grow tall through your crown, and feel a connection to the cosmos.

✶ Place your arms out to your side parallel with the earth, and bend your elbows with your hands in a fist and the thumb extended.

✶ Bring your thumbs almost to touching the tops of your shoulders and then extend the arms with the hands straight out from your shoulder sockets. Bend and straighten the elbow, inhaling your thumbs close to your shoulders and exhaling arms straight.

✶ Continue this for two to three minutes.

***

Womb Connection
Following your Fears

I recommend every pregnant person spend time at least every other day practicing relaxing. This can be meditation, taking a bath, lying in bed.... Whatever works for you and your baby.

During these relaxation times, it is inevitable that thoughts will come to your mind that feel scary. Instead of blocking these thoughts out and pretending that, if you just ignore the scary things, they won't happen, I encourage you to really explore your fears.

Follow that fear all the way to the end. What will really happen, if this fear comes to fruition? For example, what if you have a cesarean birth? Like, really... What will happen? What will you need to make this experience be okay? Do you need more support? Do you need care for your other kids? Do you need to talk to your partner about what this looks like? What do you and your baby actually need, if this fear ends up being a reality? How would you actually handle it?

Each time one of these scary thoughts comes to your mind, instead of pushing it away, follow it to the end. Shine light on it. These may not be things you really want to think about, but bringing light to your fears will help relieve them. Things usually feel less scary when we face them head-on, instead of keeping them in a what-if space.

Let your baby help you answer your what-ifs.

www.Genevamontano.com/WisdomFromTheWomb

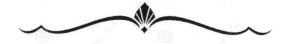

WOMB WISDOM:
JAKOTA'S STORY

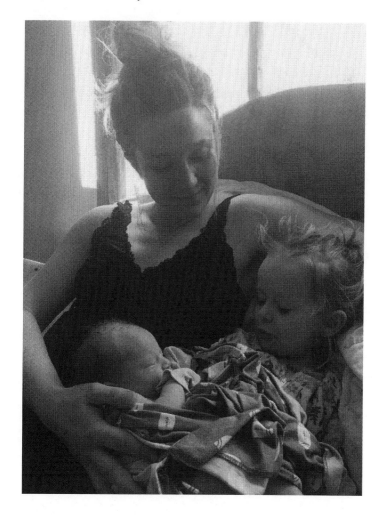

Jakota had her first baby at home with a different midwife, and a few things happened during that birth that made her question whether or not it was safe for her to have another home birth.

But her mom had home births, and she wants to be a midwife, so her heart just could not fathom having to go to the hospital to have this baby. We talked about things, and I thought she seemed like a good candidate for a home birth, as long as we did some extra monitoring and preventative nutrition therapy. I guaranteed her, as I do all parents having their second babies, this birth would be different.

Her pregnancy progressed beautifully and without complication. When we talked about trusting the baby, she expressed she wasn't sure about trusting the baby, but she was 100% on board with trusting God. She had full faith that He was holding her and her baby in His almighty hands. Who am I to argue with that?

Jakota opted not to get an ultrasound or have any other care outside of what she and I did together and the excellent care she was giving to herself. As she neared her due date, Jakota was having frequent episodes of prodromal labor. She would have slight spotting and intense contractions that never got longer, stronger, and closer together, like they do during real labor. But they would last for hours, keeping her awake, and making everyone very confused about what was happening.

At her 40-week checkup, I offered to sweep her membranes, but she still wanted to trust that her baby would pick his own birthday and keep things as natural as possible.

Her life was in upheaval those last weeks of her pregnancy. Her daughter was sick, she was sick, and the

COVID-19 virus was keeping us all in our houses, wondering about paychecks and immunity. Her husband lost his job and then thought he'd found a new one but wasn't hired due to COVID-19 hiring freezes. They weren't sure if they would be able to stay in their apartment.

In the midst of all this stress, Jakota was able to find a place of stillness where she trusted God and trusted her baby that everything was still going to be perfect and the baby would come at exactly the right time. A couple days later, Jakota called in the middle of the night because she was having bleeding she didn't understand. To me, it looked like the bleeding that comes from cervical change, but she thought it looked more like postpartum bleeding, so she asked me to come over and check her.

Her cervix told me that, indeed, there was some change happening, but I could not tell that by looking at Jakota. She was still chatty and calm, and even when she was having contractions, she was quiet. She and her husband were surprised and a little confused by how different things seemed with this baby, because she had been so vocal and needed so much support during her first labor.

The two of them did not want support from me, so I set up all my equipment and stayed on their couch, only entering their bedroom to listen to fetal heart tones. I was unsure where Jakota was at in her labor, because she wasn't showing any of the telltale signs of transition or even active labor, for that matter.

A few hours later, Jakota asked me to check her again, and she was 8 cm dilated. I called my assistant and got ready for a baby, even though I wasn't sure if there was really a baby on the way or not, with how quiet and calm Jakota was.

I asked her to get up and walk around and try to have

some stronger contractions, but Jakota was getting really tired, and this was hard for her. She had been up all night, breathing calmly through her birthing time.

The next time I went to listen to heart tones, I asked her if things were feeling different, and she told me she thought she might start pushing soon. About ten minutes later, her husband whispered out the door that I should come in. I walked in, her water broke, and the baby was born. That fast, about thirty seconds from the time I walked in the door.

Jakota wanted to catch her own baby when we talked about it prenatally, so I asked her to reach down for her baby's head, but she decided I should catch it after all—no gloves, no Chux pads, just a baby-led birth like it would have been many years ago. Wow!

Sometimes, I think I have experienced a lot of things. But this was one of the type of births I had never seen until Jakota. I read about Amish women who are completely calm and act completely normal until their baby comes out, but I have never seen it with my own eyes.

After Jakota had taken a few breaths and admired her beautiful baby boy, she said to me, "Wow, that was a supernatural birth!"

She said, with her first baby, she was prepared to be afraid and for it to be intense, and it was! With this baby, she prayed it would be easy and she would have no fear. Despite our proclamations that we believe in spiritual intervention, she and I were both surprised somehow that this prayer came true.

Oh, ye of little faith.

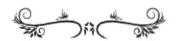

THE PREPARATIONS:
WHAT REALLY MATTERS

WHEN IT COMES TO PREPARING for birth, many people have a sort of checklist mentality, as if they are preparing for a big trip. If I check all the boxes—take the right classes, have the right baby shower, buy the right items, do the right tests, have the right nursery, create the right birth plan—then I can somehow ensure my birth will go just the way I want it to.

Unfortunately, many birthing people end up being disappointed when that day arrives and things do not go exactly as they had hoped. I find myself making a lot of promises in this book, and here's another one. I promise you your birth will *not* go exactly as you plan it. It might get close, but it won't match your expectations perfectly.

My friend Shannon is a funny example of this. I was her doula for her first birth in the hospital, and she had some qualms with how she was treated during that birth. She felt her care providers treated her differently because of her size. Even though she had an unmedicated, straightforward birth, she was told during labor that she probably would not be able to give birth vaginally, not without the help of forceps, vacuum, or even surgery. She proved them wrong and pushed her baby out like the warrior she is!

For her second birth, she chose a home birth, and I was her midwife. She had high hopes of another beautiful, natural birth but tried to be open to whatever her baby needed, even if that meant birthing in the hospital again. She had recently had her home remodeled, and her only real request for this birth was that her baby not be born in the one bathroom that had not been finished.

Her labor started at 42 weeks and, after a half a day of labor, it slowed down for a bit when she was 8 cm dilated. After some time with her husband enjoying the break in her contractions, she went to the bathroom to pee and think about what she would do next. You already know what happens next. She sat on the toilet, her water broke, she made it onto her hands and knees one step in front of the toilet, and boom! There was her baby, in the unfinished bathroom, the one thing she didn't want to happen. Baby had a different plan!

You cannot control the outcome of your birth. No matter what you do during your pregnancy, your birth will probably be a wild and unexpected ride. Whatever you think you have prepared for, those things will likely not happen, and something completely different will happen.

Most people who are hoping for a natural childbirth or even just an informed birth spend many hours researching options, talking to care providers, and taking childbirth or breastfeeding classes, doing tours, only to find out that, when they show up to have a baby, almost everything they learned goes out the window. The options they are faced with are not the ones they researched, and the information they received from care providers and tour guides does not actually apply to their situation at all.

They practice massage techniques and positions they want to try during labor. Then, when the big day arrives, when their partner touches them in the particular way that was going to be perfect, they hate it and don't want to be touched at all.

They buy the five-star-reviewed car seat and stroller, swing and monitor, and then realize the baby only wants to be on their parents' chests and never sleeps in their perfectly designed nursery.

So, why even bother preparing for birth? Sometimes, while writing this book, I myself have felt like a walking, talking contradiction. "Just trust your baby that things will be perfect, but here's all this information you don't need, because it won't change the outcome!"

What it comes down to is that your birth is important. How you feel about your birth matters, and it will affect you for the rest of your life. Ask any woman about her birth. She will have a story to tell or you will sense she has strong emotions about it. Birth changes us. You can't control it, but you can't control anything in your life!

The one thing we know for sure about life is, at the end, we will die. Knowing the outcome does not make us complacent and or uninvested in the journey of our lives. We make choices with every breath we take that will affect the quality of our lives. Some choices, we spend lots of time thinking about; some, we just follow the pack or do what we have always done; and some may come more from our heart level or gut instinct. As we make choices, we hope they will lead to the best experiences during our life, even though we know that they will not change the outcome.

No matter what choices you make, the outcome of your life will be death! It's the experiences along the way that you are affecting. Birth is just like life. The outcome is always the same. The baby comes out. The end of every single birth story is the same. The journey looks very different for each baby. I believe your baby already knows what every step of this journey looks like, but you are still the person they are relying on to make it the best journey possible for you both. The birth journey matters, and having one that you and your unborn baby enjoy and feel good about is why you are preparing.

Yes, it is actually important to prepare for your birth, even though you can't control it. But the way most pregnant people are encouraged to prepare is not working. It is not helping them be ready for the experience that lies ahead of them. Just like there is no class that teaches us how to be prepared for life or a website or book we can read that will let us know what all the options are for being a human, you can never have enough knowledge to feel like you are ready for what it actually means to be opened up in a way that allows a life to come through you.

If you were preparing to lose your virginity, you could read about sex or even practice different ways you might want to be touched while it is happening. But the way things feel while you are doing the deed likely will be quite different, and you might realize afterward that all the research you did never could have prepared you for what sex actually feels like or what you do or do not like in relation to sex. Birth and sex are similar in this way.

The good news is you don't have to do much for your baby to be born in just the right way. Knowledge and preparation might make you feel better, but your baby doesn't need it, and your baby actually has a lot more control over the course of their birth than you do. The position they choose, how much they enjoy being squeezed by your uterus, the effect baby has on your body as a foreign being growing inside—all these things will be more influential over your birthing time than the things we are generally encouraged to do to prepare for birth.

There is no book or podcast that can keep your baby's heart rate between 110-160 with good variability and accelerations. You cannot buy enough baby gadgets to keep your heart from feeling the vulnerability of parenthood. There is no genetic test that can determine what you should do if your labor is longer than you expected and you are exhausted and discouraged. There is no right combination of positions during labor that will make birth easy.

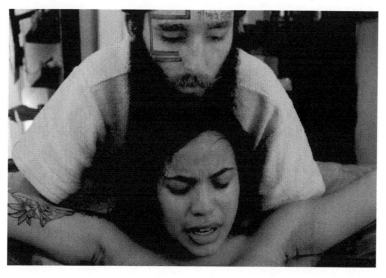

So, if you can't read or research or practice your way into the birth you want, what can you do? Well, in true contradictory form, despite what I just said a few sentences ago, it is probably important and helpful for you to know some things. I will spend some time over the next few pages giving some basics about preparing for childbirth that I have found are helpful for most people to know. It will take far less time to read these basics than it would take you to attend a childbirth class. It also might be helpful to get the feel for a few positions you might like during birth. You can find a demo of a few favorites on my website:

www.Genevamontano.com/WisdomfromtheWomb

However, most of the preparation for birth will be through spending quiet times of self-love, self-examination, and getting to know the still, small voice of your baby. In the hustle and bustle of what society tells us we need to do to be ready for a baby, I encourage you to find the time every day to connect to your baby. The wisdom and peace you are hoping to find by reading things and buying things and checking everything off the list are already within you, if you take the time to listen.

The answers you seek about your birth can never truly be provided by anyone outside of you. Your doctor doesn't actually know how the hospital staff will handle your unique birth experience. Your partner can't tell you whether or not you have a high-enough pain tolerance. Your mother's birth does not dictate how yours will go. Your midwife cannot guarantee your baby will be born at home. But you can develop a connection to yourself and to your baby that is so strong, that no matter what happens, you know everything is perfect. You can learn to trust yourself and your baby so much that you make every right decision in the perfect timing.

Sit in that perfectly designed nursery (or in the chair or bed you see yourself breastfeeding in, where your baby might actually end up spending more time), place one hand on your heart and one hand on your baby. Feel the connection of your heart to your baby's heart and listen.

Your baby will prepare you for your birth. This will happen. I believe it for you.

***

Choosing your Care Provider

Where does your baby want to be born? In this culture, most people assume they will have their baby in a hospital. It's not really even given a second thought. The media says birth happens in the hospital, and your friends and your parents probably gave birth in hospitals, and many of them tell stories that reiterate the importance of hospital birth. For many people, the hospital seems like the most reasonable place to have a baby. It is the only option with an operating room and has the most access to medicines, tests, and monitoring equipment in the case of an emergency.

If you go with this common choice, you still have options. In most hospitals, within the realm of care, there are options to birth with an OB, a family practice physician, or a midwife, plus the choice between a solo practice, a partnership, or a larger practice with many care providers.

Some people choose to go to a birthing center, in close proximity to a hospital, where there are trained personnel and specific protocols and regulations about when a person would risk out of care at the birthing center and instead have a hospital birth.

Some people feel the safest option would be to have their baby at home with a midwife supervising the birth. And some choose to have an unassisted or free birth, where they are fully in charge of their own birth, with no intervention from a trained professional.

What is the right choice for you and your baby? This is one of the most important pieces of preparing for your birth. In my experience, nothing else affects the birth experience as much as the choice of care provider. Ultimately, no person is exactly in charge of how things go. But outside of the two wills housed in your body, your care provider is really the only person who gets to call any shots. It would behoove you to find a care provider who will present you with options and honor your wishes, and who practices in a way that reflects your values.

No matter where you birth, you might consider hiring a doula. A doula is a professional birth support person. They are trained in the ins and outs of childbirth and early parenthood. They are also people who have been caregivers all their life. They love supporting birthing people.

Having a doula takes the pressure off of you and your partner to know everything about birth. A doula can help you to know what questions to ask or if you are receiving all the information you could about decisions you might have to make. Doulas can suggest comfort measures when appropriate. They can encourage your partner to take a break when needed. Most of all, they remind the birthing person of their own magic and power. They hold space for them to be strong, to ask for what they need, to connect to the baby, and to create a loving container for all people involved in the birth. Your doula does not provide any medical care but will be a very supportive part of any birth team. Their goal is for you to look back on your birth as a positive experience, no matter what that looks like.

Obstetricians are trained surgeons. They have been through medical school, and their training teaches them to keep an eye out for things that could go wrong during birth and then to fix those things. Family practice doctors also go through medical school and have some surgical training, but not to the same extent as an OB. They try to keep the whole family in mind, thinking of what is best for the birthing person, the baby, and their family, as decisions are made during care.

The midwife's model of care teaches that birth is normal and to look for signs of everything being normal.[6] If things are outside the realm of normal, they generally call in the support of a physician, who has more training on things that are outside of normal ranges. Within the sisterhood of midwives, there are some who do most or all of their schooling in hospital-based settings, who may take a more medical approach to birth, and some who practice a more traditional midwifery, with fewer protocols and routine procedures. This is also true of various physicians.

Those who choose unassisted birth act as their own care providers and arrange the cares that are important to them as they see fit.

Every care provider comes with their own set of experiences, knowledge, beliefs, and protocols. There is no such thing as one size fits all, and you can find great care or crappy care from any of these models. Does one of these models speak to you or your baby? (Ask the baby.)

The obvious benefit of being at a hospital is the proximity to advanced equipment, drugs, and trained specialists. Drawbacks might include restrictive or unnecessary protocols, increased levels of intervention, increased reliance on technology, and lack of relationship with care providers.

When you walk into many hospitals, you immediately become a patient, a sick person who needs to be treated, instead of a warrior goddess, accessing your inner power to create life. In most cases, you will be monitored for at least twenty minutes (often longer), asked to put on a hospital gown, asked 1.2 million questions about everything from your diet and spiritual preferences to your health history to whether or not you brought a wedding ring with you, and have blood drawn and an IV placed—all before you really have your feet under you in the room, especially if you labor at home until you are in active labor (which is recommended). Most hospitals have policies about consuming food, the acceptable length of labor, monitoring, where in the room you can birth, when the umbilical cord is cut, when baby has to go to NICU, how often baby eats, where baby sleeps, and many other things. Each of these protocols, while in place to keep you and baby safe, can create obstacles when it comes to having the birth you may envision or may feel your baby wants.

Birth centers are a great option for people who don't want to be in a hospital with the routine interventions but feel safer being cared for in a location other than their home. Birth centers have protocols in place to make a smooth transfer of care to the hospital, if the pregnancy or the birth become risky—for example, if the birthing person's blood pressure becomes elevated, or if there is meconium present when the bag of waters ruptures. They have emergency drugs and equipment readily available, but the goal is to never have to use those things. If they are used, a trip to the hospital may ensue. Birth centers are usually peaceful and homey, and the family stays for several hours after the birth before they drive home with their new baby.

At a homebirth, the midwife brings to your house all or most of the same equipment that the birth center has. She stays with you from active labor until a few hours after the birth (more or less, depending on the midwife). The same person who did your prenatal care is usually the person who will catch your baby. You have developed a relationship with her, and she has a vested interest in the outcome of your birth, just like you. She still cannot control the outcome, but she does usually care deeply about it.

Many people in our culture do not consider home birth as an option. But when we look back at human history, people have only been going to the hospital to give birth for 100 years. This is a very short amount of time. A blip on the map of human history. It's a fad. Women have always given birth at home, with the support of midwives. If birth outside of a hospital was extremely dangerous, the human race would not still exist; our species would have died out, if birth didn't work correctly.

You might have heard the theory about the human fetal head being too big for the female human pelvis and that this is a design or evolutionary flaw. This is called the obstetric dilemma, and it's a real thing some people believe in, even though babies come through female pelvises every day. Even with giant heads, somehow birth still works, and we have managed to populate the Earth with almost eight billion people, so something must be working!

Home birth is usually far less interrupted than births that require the birthing person to get in the car and get situated in a new location. For those people who want a natural birth, having less interruptions means the body has more chance to do what it is physiologically designed to do.

I obviously have a bias for home birth. After witnessing over 200 at home, 300 in the hospital, and dozens at birth centers, I feel strongly that home birth is a good option for low-risk women.[7] (Side note: if you want a good laugh, the comedian Jim Gaffigan talks about home birth in his special, *Mr. Universe*; it's a funny but true look at this option. For something more serious, *The Business of Being Born, Orgasmic Birth* and *Why Not Home* are interesting documentaries about your choices.)

Some families decide they feel comfortable birthing without the support of anyone. They gather the supplies and skills needed to have a baby in their home without the support of a trained professional. Free birth can be a beautiful option. Most babies do come on their own, needing very little assistance from anyone, when the baby is in charge and the birthing body and mind are prepared and open to the experience. I admittedly do not have experience with free birth, because if I am present at a birth, it is no longer unassisted. I have had a few families who worked with me for their first or second babies and then chose to have a free birth with subsequent babies, after moving to a new location where they could not find a provider they felt comfortable with. Their births were reportedly uncomplicated and magical. The Free Birth Society and Indie Birth might be good websites to explore, if this option appeals to you and your baby.

The drawback of birthing at home or a birthing center, with or without assistance, is, of course, if something goes wrong, you are farther away from the medical help you might need.

True emergencies in birth are exceedingly rare. There are almost always warning signs ahead of time that something isn't quite right, and a skilled birth-keeper will almost always notice those things. Plus, your intuition, your body, or your baby will warn you. You are the expert on your body and your baby. You will know if something is not perfect within you. Learning to listen to your unborn baby's whispers (and especially not ignoring when the whispers become sirens) is a skill and a gift you can develop, one that will serve you well as a parent and as a human.

No matter where you choose to birth your baby, ultimately you are responsible for your experience. No doctor or midwife can save you from the experience you are going to have, though they may try, and the experience might then look different. Either way, you are going to have an experience. Your job is to breathe, listen to the still, small voices, trust, and make the choices that create the most positive experience for you and your baby.

If you choose a care provider who has a lot of tools that are designed as a safety net in case things go wrong, then they will be using those tools to examine closely if things are going wrong. When we look hard enough for things that are going wrong, we are likely to find them! If you are hoping for a natural birth with minimal interventions, then going to a care provider at a hospital where they are required to use these tools as a safety net might not be the best option. It is important to spend time throughout your pregnancy checking in with yourself and your baby to determine how you really want your birth to look.

If your vision for your birth is to be in a bathtub in the dark with candles, undisturbed, with your partner catching the baby and the two of you admiring the baby silently and peacefully, alone in your own little world... That is probably not going to happen at any hospital. I have been to so many beautiful, amazing hospital births. But not one has ever looked like that. There are monitors and IVs and people (so many people) and lights and beeping machines... All things that are there as a safety net. If you don't want those things, then you really can't birth at a hospital. It's not a judgement, just the truth.

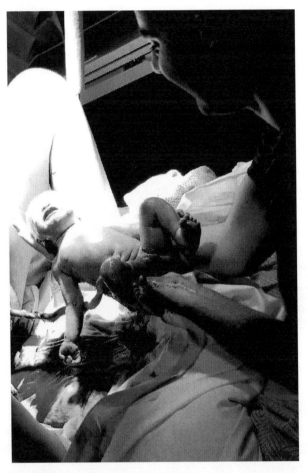

I recently attended a birth at the hospital where the baby came quickly with no fuss or trouble. The dad caught the baby with no care provider in the room, and I guided him to place baby onto mom's belly. The amount of people who ran in after this birth would make you think there was an emergency. So many tools, so much energy and anxiety—for a birth that had already completed uneventfully!

No matter what your care provider says about how supportive they are of natural childbirth, if your vision of birth does not include the safety net tools, you cannot have your ideal birth at a hospital. It's like walking into McDonald's and telling them you want a pizza. They can do their best and put some ketchup and cheese slices on a bun for you, but they can never make you a pizza. Not because they are terrible people who want to ruin your meal. They just don't have the right ingredients.

If you choose a care provider who has a very high cesarean rate or induction rate, you are more likely to be induced or have a cesarean, no matter how nice they are or how much you like them! There are very nice, supportive, intelligent care providers out there whose lived experiences have made them feel safer with induction and surgical birth. If you want to be induced or have a cesarean, you should choose one of these providers! If you think you can have a candlelit water birth with them, you could be fooling yourself. Or maybe they are trying to fool you.

It may be taboo to say this, but care providers want your money. They will often say whatever they think you want to hear, in order to have you as a patient and bill your insurance. I encourage you to check in with yourself often throughout your prenatal care. Is your care provider offering the experience you had hoped to have? Do you feel safe? Do you feel supported? Do you feel heard? When you get quiet and check in with your baby, does this care provider and the care you are receiving resonate with them? If it does, wonderful! You are in the right place, and you have taken one of the most important and powerful steps toward having the sacred birth you desire and deserve. If not, what is missing? Do you need to look into other providers or just have a heart to heart with yours?

It is never too late to change care providers. At any point, you could decide to find a new provider, and unless you are in a very small town and are unable or unwilling to travel, you can find another provider who is willing to take your money. Honestly, most care providers are so busy, they barely notice if someone switches care. Sad as it may be, if you aren't feeling a magical connection with your provider, you, your birth, and your baby are probably not overly important to them. There are people who switch to a new provider or even home birth care after 41 weeks. There are people who decide at the last minute to have a free birth. There are people who decide during labor that they feel safer at a hospital than at home. It is never too late to change your mind. (Unless your baby is coming out; then, it might be too late.)

Checking in with yourself and your baby early and often will bring the added benefit of having more time with care that feels right and allows you to settle in and gain comfort and familiarity with the new provider, if you decide you do need to make a change. It feels scary to change providers. Really scary. Humans are most comfortable with the things they are familiar with. Many people stay with a care provider they do not love or trust because it feels too daunting to make that change. They feel like they are making a fuss, being too demanding, making waves. We are creatures of habit.

You have the option of staying in your comfort zone. But if the baby's quiet whispers are telling you this is not the right fit for you, that you cannot have the sacred birth you desire with this provider, I hope you will listen. You are a goddess creating life! Have you ever heard of a goddess who sat quietly and just let things happen around her so she didn't make waves or bother anyone? Seriously, inside of you at this moment is the same power that created the universe. You are magical and miraculous. Create all the waves! Storm and thrash and light fires! Burn some stuff down, if that's what it takes! This is your baby's birth! The only time this baby will ever be born. How do they want it to be?

***

WOMB CONNECTION
CHANNELING THE MOTHER GODDESS

Durga is the fierce mother goddess in the Hindu religion. She is the epitome of powerful and doesn't let anyone stop her on her path. She rides a lion and has eight arms, yielding weapons and flowers. She slayed demons that no one else could. It is said that meditating on Durga can bring forth warrior-like strength and protective compassion—that mama-bear energy.

When you bring her energy into your inner world, she can empower you and guide you through conflict and drama and help you let go of the illusions and fears that hold you back.

Durga Kriya 1

* Stand with your feet wide apart, toes pointing outward, and your arms up overhead, fingers spread wide in star pose. Shout "*Maha!*"

* Gather all the power of Durga into your fists as you bring your elbows in next to your ribs, fists facing up, elbows bent at a 90-degree angle. Knees bend to a 90-degree angle, as well, into goddess pose.

* Bring tension into every muscle of your body as you come down into your womb energy and roar "*Durga*" like the mama bear you are.

* Repeat this, moving from star—"*Maha*"—to goddess with warrior arms—"*Durga*"—for one to two

minutes. Feel the power of the protective, ferocious mother grow in every cell of your body.

Durga Kriya 2-

* Grab an imaginary spear in your right hand, and lift it up overhead. Lift your left leg, and imagine your fears standing next to you.

* With a mighty yell, shouting *"Durga"* or any primitive noise that comes up for you, drop your weight onto your left leg as you power the spear through your fears. Don't be shy. Let your throat chakra experience being completely open as you allow Durga's fierce energy to slay your demons.

* Repeat five to seven times on each side.

www.Genevamontano.com/WisdomFromTheWomb

***

PREPARING YOUR BODY FOR BIRTH

PREPARING YOUR BODY for birth is wise. Your uterus has to grow from the size of a pear to the size of a watermelon. This growth changes just about everything else in your body. There's more pressure on your lower extremities. It is more difficult to breathe, and your stomach and intestines have to find room to do their work. Just sitting on the couch while you are pregnant burns more calories than the average man needs while he is working out. Your heart pumps more blood, your liver processes more hormones, and your bones support more weight. There is so much going on in your body!

Throughout history, women have been honored during pregnancy. They were encouraged to luxuriate in the magical work of creation happening inside their bodies. They sometimes continued doing other work, because pregnancy is not an illness and pregnant people are still capable of doing normal activities. However, they were seen as being in a sacred state and their wishes were revered. If a pregnant person was tired, they would be encouraged to rest. If they were hungry, they were encouraged to eat.

Clocks did not have the same significance to ancient

peoples that they do to twenty-first-century people. Being in a delicate state lent even more toward honoring the body's needs at any given time, rather than waiting for a clock to say it's time to eat or wake up or go to sleep or take time to connect with the baby.

For most pregnant people in America today, it is almost impossible to honor ourselves the way our bodies and souls expect to be honored while we are creating life. Therefore, it is up to you and your support circle to set very specific goals and boundaries on what you want your daily care and routines to look like while you are pregnant. At a bare minimum, I would encourage you to check in with your baby several times a day, to see what they need at that precise moment. Are they tired? Do they need more calories or more rest? Do they like it when you move, because it rocks them to sleep? Do they just need a moment to feel close to the only person they know on this Earth?

Pregnant people need to eat more often than they usually think. In early pregnancy, morning sickness is often related to a blood sugar drop caused by not eating all night long. One way to help with this is to have a high-protein snack right before bed, and if you wake up to pee in the middle of the night, see if you can toss back a couple almonds or other protein-rich snack. Before you get out of bed in the morning, have another handful.

You might need to experiment to figure out which foods your baby likes and which they have an aversion to. But you have to eat. Find something you can eat. For pregnant people who struggle more severely with nausea, I recommend they set a timer for every ninety minutes to two hours, to remind them to eat. If you get hungry, then your blood sugar has already dropped and your baby has already felt the effect of a mini-fast. Try to eat before you get hungry. Babies are very resourceful, and they will take from your body what they need. That leaves your body at risk of deficiencies during a time when you need all the nourishment possible.

Cravings for high-carb foods and sweets increase for many people during pregnancy. Consuming a lot of sugar can throw off your microbiome as well as raise blood pressure, cause heartburn, UTIs, yeast infections, swelling, placental degradation, inflammation, headaches and a wealth of other not-so-great symptoms.

While I generally recommended you listen to your body and your baby and honor what they need, sometimes the sugar craving is simply an energy craving. When our bodies need energy, they look for the quickest form of energy possible, which is carbs and sugar. However, sustained energy is created by protein. Our bodies also think of sweets and carbs as a reward and are looking for positive reinforcement and love. Is there a way you can give your body and your baby the energy and love they are looking for without indulging in sugar?

Try paying close attention to exactly why you are craving sugar. Is it emotional? Or because you went too long without calories? Or does your baby want some natural sweetness? Is it actually a Snickers bar that you need or could an apple do the trick? Just ask and notice, before you partake, and maybe even try a handful or a spoonful of something with protein before you indulge in the Snickers. See if that changes your craving at all.

Most pregnant people need at least 100 ounces of water per day, but those of us who live at high altitude or in dry or hot climates or who are doing a lot of physical work or sitting in buildings that have heaters or air conditioners blowing on them regularly, or who are experiencing stress in any way might need more water. (This probably includes you!) I live in Colorado. It is very dry here, and we are at a fairly high altitude. I find that most people are walking around dehydrated, even the ones who are not pregnant.

If our electrolytes get off balance for any reason, such as vomiting, traveling, or having a few days of dehydration, then we need to replenish electrolytes as well as water. If you feel like you are drinking all the time and just peeing it straight out but not actually getting hydrated, this is probably why. If you are having muscle cramps or a lot of Braxton Hicks contractions or headaches or dizziness, electrolyte imbalance could be the culprit there, as well. You might need to add some broth or diluted Gatorade or cucumber water or Emergen-C or some other form of electrolytes to your daily fluid intake. Again, check in with yourself and with your baby after you drink the electrolytes, and notice how you feel.

We often only notice when we feel bad, but try to start to pay attention to what makes you feel really good! Talk to your baby, and tell them everything you're putting in your mouth is for them. Every bite you take is nourishing your cells as well as theirs and setting them up for a beautiful birth and a beautiful future.

One of the primary fears I hear about from pregnant people is the fear of tearing during birth. Being well-hydrated and well-nourished, with lots of protein, healthy fats, and vitamins A, C, and E, can help your tissues be pliable, so they stretch exactly the way they are designed to during your birthing process, instead of tearing. These nutrients can also build a nice, strong amniotic sac that doesn't rupture before labor begins.

Just to reiterate—sugar, which is also a main ingredient in all processed foods, increases your likelihood of tearing, as well as your likelihood of having any disease of pregnancy. (This includes pregnancy-induced hypertension, pre-eclampsia, gestational diabetes, even testing positive for group-B strep.)

If you do still tear, you will heal more quickly if your tissues are as healthy as possible beforehand. This is also important for women who have a surgical birth. Recovery is easier for everyone, but particularly for women who have undergone a major surgery, when hydration and nourishment during pregnancy are on point. Babies are also more stable after birth when they have been given all the water and nutrients their bodies need in utero. How your body is nourished during pregnancy will make a difference in how you and your baby feel during your birthing time, how quickly you heal and your baby transitions into this Earth-side life.

Many pregnant people find themselves feeling fatigued, which can be from a lack of minerals such as iron or magnesium, or it can be from a lack of cell-building proteins. The best source of minerals is leafy green vegetables, and there is protein in almost every naturally found food. Broccoli is super-high in protein. Grains. Of course, animal products, but if you are averse to animal products or choose not to partake in them for other reasons, it's still recommended to shoot for 80-100 grams of protein per day, in order to support your body as it is building a new human.

Of course, fatigue could also be caused by working too hard or not sleeping enough. Our culture does not generally support rest—we are taught that we are useful humans if we are productive and hard-working.

Growing a new human is productive and hard enough. Give yourself some grace, and see what you can take off your plate. Can you work less hours or have someone help with the kids or the house? Can you stay in bed all day every Saturday? Can you go to bed earlier? You might have to get creative or sacrifice a few things in order to make this happen. You are worth it! You deserve to rest. You are doing good work and creating a cultural shift and a better world for your baby by making yourself a priority.

If you aren't sleeping well, see if you can determine why. Is it your mind or your body keeping you awake? If it is your body, a high-protein snack before bed or a calcium-magnesium supplement could help. A warm bath, chamomile tea, some loving touch. What do you and your baby need to be comfortable? More pillows? A bedtime yoga routine? See if your care provider or doula have any ideas. If it is your mind, sometimes journaling before bed or when you wake up helps your mind relax. Listening to a guided meditation or something like *Hypnobabies* or hypnobirthing can help. Can you talk to your baby about what is keeping you awake?

If sleeping at night continues to be an issue it will be important that you take naps. Just like with food, it's important to enter into your birthing and postpartum time in a non-deficient state. Again, get creative—what can you set up and who can you call on to help you with other things, so you can get some sleep. Pregnancy is a great time to build your community of support people. When someone asks if you need anything, say yes! You are worthy of love and support. Your baby needs you to learn to receive.

Birth is like a marathon, so preparing your body to run a marathon is also recommended. If a person trains for a marathon and only gets halfway through then has to walk or even be carried the rest of the way, they usually feel pretty good about the effort they put in and how far they made it. The person who never tries may always have regrets. The person who never even wanted to run a marathon but did anyway might regret trying or might still feel proud of themselves that they tried something they didn't think they could do. The same is true with birth and with choosing to have a natural childbirth.

No matter your stance on marathons, it is important to exercise during pregnancy! I don't know of anyone who just gets up one day and decides to run a marathon and completes it successfully. They have either trained previously or are currently in training when they decide to do this. You will need to prepare your physical body for the marathon of birth. Even if your birth is a sprint, your body needs the physical preparation of exercising.

Research shows that babies who grow in the womb of someone who exercises are healthier at birth.[8] They are better able to regulate their body temperature, blood sugar levels, even their emotions. Babies who are exposed to regular exercise actually cry less! They have become accustomed to experiencing some stress and then also experiencing the good feeling that comes after that stress, in the form of endorphins, when the stress is exercise-induced.

Your baby wants you to exercise. I don't even need you to ask your baby if this is true. I already know it is. You can ask your baby what kind of exercise they like the best or what time of day they prefer, but unless it's a health risk for you, your baby wants you to exercise. If you have been living a sedentary lifestyle before you got pregnant, it is definitely not recommended to start a new strenuous exercise routine. But some walks or some prenatal yoga or swimming are good and healthy for most everyone.

It is recommended to exercise for thirty minutes a day or an hour every other day. Your heart rate should be elevated to a point where you cannot sing a song. However, if you cannot hold a conversation, then you are working too hard. Talk and sing to your baby while you are exercising! If you can still sing, work harder! If you can't talk, take it down a notch.

If you are unable to get into an exercise routine, just moving regularly throughout the day also has benefits. Chasing around a toddler or cleaning do have benefits. Getting up from your desk and dancing with the baby in your belly for a few minutes or even walking to the bathroom and stretching every hour counts!

Part of the benefit of exercise is also the good feelings and the hormones that accompany them, so I recommend finding something that brings you joy. Do you like walking in the sunshine or being able to speak to other pregnant people at prenatal exercise classes? Does being in the water take away all the worries of your day while you are swimming? Or does being in nature remind you where you come from? Do you want to try belly dancing or just a good old-fashioned booty shake in your living room? Whatever it is, you should notice you feel really good when you're done. Check in with your baby. I bet they feel really good, as well. They might even give you a few extra minutes of sleep before head-butting your bladder.

There is an added benefit of exercise that is not physical. Birth is really hard work. And most of it is not physical work.

Most of it is mental. Most birthing people, at some point during their journey, feel like they cannot keep going, like birth is just too difficult. Some even feel like they might die. Birth is a rite of passage. Pam England talks about how birthing people have to come to the point of surrendering all that they are, in order to give birth. Her books, *Birthing from Within* and *Ancient Maps for Modern Birth*, are amazing at addressing this and are highly recommended for any pregnant person, but particularly those who have had a previous traumatic birth.

During birth, you will likely be pushed to your limits. Knowing how to keep going after you have been pushed, after you have reached your limit, is one of the most important things you can do to prepare. Getting up and exercising sucks. Most people do not love it. Do it anyway!! If you want to have the best chances at a vaginal birth, or if you want an easier recovery and a healthier baby, seriously, just do it!

Yes, I know you are growing a baby and you are tired. I promise, if you just do it, you will feel better. If you hate it and do it anyway and then afterward realize how much better you feel, this will help you get through birth. It will be in your muscle memory to do the things that are hard and that you don't want to do.

Sometimes, we get to a point in our workout where we don't think we can keep going, we think we have reached the maximum we can give. But then, when we keep going, we realize we are actually doing just fine and have a lot more to give than we originally thought. Practice doing something that you don't really want to do or don't think you are capable of. It will be immensely helpful when it comes time for your baby to be born.

You are stronger than you know, and you have what it takes—both to work out and to birth your baby. When you start to feel tired, dig deep, and ask your baby to help you. They will give you energy when you feel like you're done. Draw on the strength of all the babies who have been born before yours. All the women who have birthed before you.

You are supported. You are surrounded by love. Let that love and support give you strength and energy. The universe itself has got your back. You have everything you need. You've got this.

***

WOMB CONNECTION
KRIYAS

I have already described a few kriyas in previous chapters. Kriya yoga is one of my favorite techniques for practicing pushing your limits. Sometimes in prenatal yoga classes, kriyas are called "keep-ups." This is a Kundalini Yoga technique that has been scientifically proven to shift patterns stored in cells.

These techniques can offer a great opportunity to push your limits, because it's often also very difficult to keep going when you do them. But they will teach you that you have what it takes to keep going.

Check in with your baby, and see which one of these kriyas is the most relevant for you and your sweet baby. Do one or more every day for two to three minutes. When it gets hard, keep going!

If your baby enjoys doing kriya yoga, my favorite book to get more of this powerful goodness is *Bountiful, Beautiful, Blissful* by Gurmukh.

Releasing anger and grief:

* ✶ Sit with a strong spine.

* ✶ As you inhale through the nose, outstretch the arms upward to a 45-degree angle, opening the palms.

* ✶ Open your heart and gaze slightly upward.

* ✶ As you exhale strongly out of the mouth (making the sound *shhhh*), draw the elbows in and down, and create fists with the thumbs tucked in that face in

toward the body. The movement is very quick, and the energy focused.

We store grief and anger in our lungs and liver. This movement can help release stuck emotions. This also massages the lymph nodes in the armpits and increases energy.

Heart-opening kriya:

- ✳ Sit with a strong spine.

- ✳ Bring your hands in front of your face, palms facing one another about six inches apart, elbows at a 90-degree angle.

- ✳ Exhale sharply as you pull the arms apart from one another with force, as though you are hitting imaginary walls with your forearms on each side of you. With each exhale, imagine you are moving all obstacles that keep your heart closed.

Balancing the masculine and feminine:

- ✳ Sit with a strong spine.

- ✳ Bring your hands up to your shoulders, thumbs in front and four fingers on the back of your shoulders, with your arms parallel to the floor.

- ✳ As you inhale, turn to the left, and as you exhale, turn to the left. You can start slowly, to warm up your spine.

- ✳ After a moment, do this double-time, and take your baby on a ride.

www.Genevamontano.com/WisdomFromTheWomb

***

Physical Fitness

Diet, hydration, and exercise are the basic building blocks of a healthy pregnancy. But to achieve the most successful chances of having the birth you and your baby desire, we want to think about the details of your physical body and not just the basics. So, let's dig in a little bit deeper.

Babies come in all shapes and sizes and affect the womb they are carried in in all different ways. If you line up ten pregnant people next to one another, some look like they are carrying basketballs under their shirt, straight out front. Others will carry lower, others higher. Some will carry through the breadth of their torsos, and some even look like they're carrying more in their butts. All of this is normal. What is not normal is a lot of discomfort!

We have been taught to believe that pregnancy is just a time where you have to accept you will feel bad. That is not true! Remember: you are a goddess, and you are meant to be nourished, honored, and feel amazing during this time. Yes, you will feel very different as a human grows inside you. But if something feels wrong, it probably is.

Your care provider may or may not agree with this philosophy, so you might need to talk to alternative health providers or a doula to get ideas of how to relieve the discomforts of pregnancy. Our bodies always want to find alignment and perfect health. If we give them the opportunity to do so, they will.

If you are feeling a lot of discomfort in your upper body—shortness of breath, difficulty breathing, loss of appetite, heartburn, nausea, vomiting, etc.—this could be because you are carrying your baby high. Conversely, babies who are carried low can cause things like hemorrhoids, varicose veins, swelling, or hip and lower back pain. These are all things many people consider normal in pregnancy, but they do not have to be.

If there's a lot of tension in your lower belly, underneath your baby, this might make it difficult for baby to find the right location in your belly to sink down low enough. The reverse is true for babies that are carried low: you might have tension or adhesions in your upper abdomen or diaphragm. Again, try talking to your baby. See if you can feel what position they are in, touch your body, and feel if there's anything in your tissues that is keeping baby from finding the optimal location, right in the center of your body.

Massage your tissues all around your pelvis and your pubic bone up your waist and under your ribs. Take your time, and let your tissues talk to you and tell you which areas might need some love and attention. Place your hands on your belly, and ask baby to come into the perfect position— head down, chin tucked, spine toward your belly.

You might reach out to a prenatal massage therapist or physical therapist or chiropractor, to help you get your body back into balance. Any slight misalignment in your body can affect your birth greatly and not just your pregnancy.

Birth is designed to work in a very specific way. The baby chooses to enter your pelvis in most cases, with its head facing one hip or the other. The shape of their head only fits through the shape of most female pelvises on that angle. However, in order for the head to exit through the pelvic outlet it has to turn to face the front or the back. Then it has to turn again to get the shoulders through the pelvic outlet. You don't have to think about any of this while you are in labor—your body and your baby will do the work. You can assist this process by having your baby in an optimal position before labor begins. For most people, this optimal position is head down with the back of the baby's head on the left side of the birthing pelvis. This position is called LOA, left occiput anterior, meaning the baby's occiput bone, the back of their skull, is on the left front side of the pregnant body.

Most babies will turn head-down by about 32-33 weeks, as their head gets heavier and gravity pulls it down. If, at 32 weeks, your baby has not moved to a head-down position, you might start thinking about ways to encourage your baby to make the move.

I always recommend starting with the least interventive techniques, and then pulling out the big guns if they are needed.

Start by talking to your baby. Let them know there is a very comfortable, head-shaped bowl down at the bottom of your abdomen, and the door to their new life is also down there. That being said, if your baby feels unsafe or like something is upside down in your life, they might feel more inclined to stay in a breech position, with their head close to your heart and in a position that helps them feel farther away from the door. If your baby is breech, you might spend some time asking yourself and your baby if anything feels upside down in your life, or if exiting feels unsafe, and make some solid plans to correct this.

It is helpful to visualize your baby in a head-down position and to see images of babies in the correct position. You could put a picture on your mirror or as the screensaver on your phone, of a baby in the optimal position, head down with its chin tucked to its chest and hands down away from its face.

Spinningbabies.com is a fantastic website that talks about body alignment and turning a baby into the optimal position. I highly recommend exploring this website; consider doing their daily and weekly activities throughout your pregnancy. Doing these activities gives you time to connect with your baby and visualize their birth going exactly as it should.

Beyond being head down, it is also ideal if your baby is positioned with their back toward the front side of your body. Most babies don't actually turn to this position until you are in labor, but their back will usually be just to one side or the other of the front of your belly, with their chin tucked to their chest and hands down away from their face. This position allows the smallest diameter of the baby's head to present at the widest diameter of your pelvis. If baby's head is facing the other direction (occiput posterior) or even slightly tilted to one side or the other (asynclitic), it allows a much larger diameter of the head to present into the pelvis. It is absolutely possible in many cases to birth an asynclitic or occiput posterior baby vaginally. But it is a lot more difficult.

On average, a baby who is not in the optimal position will have a labor about ten hours longer than a baby that is optimally positioned. During those ten hours, there are usually more contractions, because the body is working hard to move the baby into an optimal position. Each contraction is more painful, because the baby's head is pressing in a different, non-optimal way on your bones. One of the most important things you can do to have a smooth and efficient labor is to spend time prenatally, encouraging your baby into an optimal position.[9]

This is done mostly by gravity. The heaviest part of the

baby is the head; the back of their head and the upper spine specifically are the heaviest. So, wherever you are sitting, lying, or standing, think about where gravity is pulling your baby. If you often kick back with your feet up into a soft, comfy couch, then gravity is pulling the back of the head and the spine down toward the Earth, which is encouraging baby into an occiput posterior position. If you sit with your legs crossed or in a very imbalanced posture on one hip or the other, your baby is likely to enter the pelvis in an asynclitic position, with their head cocked off to one side or the other.

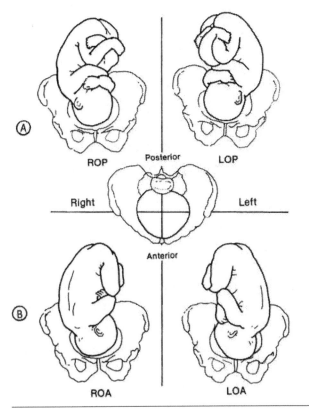

The ideal way to spend the majority of your time for the most efficient birth is to have both of your sitz bones evenly on whatever surface you are sitting on and your belly button pointing straight ahead or down. I highly encourage you to look further into optimal fetal positioning.

Amazingly, most pregnant people also find that they are much more comfortable when they shift their posture to encourage baby into the optimal position. Back aches and sore hips begin to disappear when their bodies are aligned. When they start to pay closer attention, they also notice that their babies seem more comfortable. Pay attention to your baby's kicks. What do they mean? Is your baby trying to move into a better position? Or are they just stretching their legs? Imagine if you were in a tight space with a kink in your neck for weeks. You would probably be hoping that someone would notice you need a little help to get in a better position!

Today, I had someone come in for her appointment who was complaining of pain in her pubic bone and her hips when she walked. We discussed different ways she might be able to relieve this for quite some time, before I put my hands on her belly. When I touched her belly, I realized her baby was already lodged into her pelvis at 32 weeks. Baby's head was putting unnecessary pressure on her pubic bone in a weird position, and it was causing her pain.

We released the tissues under her ribs around the top of her uterus, so baby had some room to move up into her upper abdomen. Then, when I gently lifted her lower belly up with my fingertips near her pubic bone, baby came up out of her pelvis, and she felt an immediate relief. It allowed her baby to find some freedom of movement and a more comfortable position. She was so ecstatic when she got up off my table. The pain she had been feeling from a non-optimal fetal position was completely gone.

I will reiterate: you do not have to be in pain just because you are pregnant. Pain is a warning signal that something is wrong, and just being pregnant is not something wrong. Expect things to feel different, but if you are in pain, chances are your baby is also uncomfortable, and there are measures you can take to help both of you feel better. Webster-certified chiropractors are a great resource, as are Mayan abdominal massage practitioners, and physical therapists specifically trained in prenatal techniques (my favorite is the Institute for Birth Healing). Find someone who can help you get out of pain. It will benefit your body, your baby, and your birth.

All that being said—some babies pick a different position for birth, and they are born just perfectly in positions that care providers might think are more difficult or sometimes near impossible to birth in. If you are tuned into your baby, they might tell you something completely different than what I have outlined. Your baby has its own unique needs, preferences, and plan for its birth. Trust what you feel from your baby. Let them guide you.

***

It could be really tempting to start judging yourself for the physical choices you have made thus far in your pregnancy. Maybe you had a little too much to drink before you found out you were pregnant, while you were out with the girls. Maybe you really love McDonald's French fries, and you have had some every day since you got pregnant. Maybe it's the only thing you could eat that didn't make you throw up in the first trimester. Maybe you've really gotten into *Call the Midwife* and *Working Moms* on Netflix; it's just really hard to focus on your baby, when these TV babies have so much going on that you want to pay attention to. Sometimes, lying on the couch just seems like a lot better idea than going for a walk. It's okay. I get it.

We also know that the physical and emotional are intricately intwined, and when we feel stress and anxiety, or sadness and guilt, we are bathing our babies in the same hormones that flow through our own veins. During pregnancy, we have a tendency to stress over the stress we feel and feel guilty about every negative thought that crosses our mind, because we know it can affect our babies.

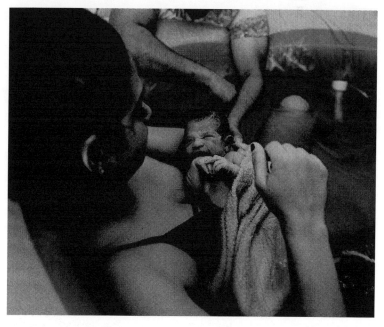

Give yourself grace and think about yourself the way your baby thinks about you. Have you seen the way a new baby looks at their mother? From the moment a baby is born, they have the most incredible, forgiving love. That baby does not care one bit what happened during their birth or while they were growing inside. As soon as they are on your chest, all covered in vernix and amniotic fluid, and they open their eyes for the first time, they are searching for that one connection, the heartbeat they knew in utero, the eyes and face that match that heartbeat. The baby is searching for its mother.

This baby has never been born before, not in this body, not in this time or dimension. Whatever experience they get, they are happy to have that experience; it is the experience they were hoping and waiting for. Your baby will forgive all of your mistakes and all the things you did knowingly. Your baby thinks you are the most magical of all creatures. You hold them and feed them and let them listen to the rhythm of your heartbeat and your breath. Your touch, your voice, your thoughts and feelings, and the chemicals you produce are all your baby has ever known.

Let go of any blame you are feeling and any guilt for choices you have made up to this point. Your baby doesn't care, and they are the only one that really matters. Even if you eat a 100% organic diet, exercise daily, think only pure thoughts, go to bed early, and otherwise live the perfect life, your baby is still getting environmental toxins and whatever else might have built up in your body over the years.

Remember: your baby picked you to be their parent. That being said, as you move forward, full of grace and love for yourself, try to take a small pause before you make decisions about your food and lifestyle. Think about this beautiful creature growing inside of you. Think about their tiny toenails and their soft skin, their growing organs and the neurons forming connections in their brain. What does your baby want to eat? What chemicals does your baby want to experience? What can you do to produce more of those chemicals?

No guilt or shame if, one day, you eat ice cream straight out of the container with a fork. Just a pause before you open the freezer, so you are doing it with full consent of your own free will and your baby's still, small voice.

***

WOMB CONNECTION
PELVIC BOWL SWEEP

Modified from *The Wild Feminine* by Tami Lynn Kent

* Let your eyes close.

* Feel all the areas of your body that are making contact with something. Your bottom, your back, your feet. Feel yourself being supported.

* Feel the energy of the Earth drawing up into your body, and see that energy swirling inside your pelvis.

* Reach your crown toward the sky, and feel yourself drawing energy down from the cosmos. Draw this energy down through your head, through your chest and abdomen, and allow it to mix with the energy from the Earth in your pelvis.

* See the energy of the Earth and the energy of the cosmos co-mingling and infusing your baby and your body with energy.

* Visualize your pelvis as a bowl. Just notice what this bowl looks like. Is it deep or shallow? Is it tilted to one side or the other? Does it have a color or a pattern? Are there any cracks or blemishes?

* Now, imagine yourself cleaning out your bowl. Use the energy from the Earth and the sky. Use

whatever other tools you need. Work your way around to the inside and the outside of the bowl. If there are any parts of your bowl that do not want to be cleaned, just let them know you see them and continue cleaning the other parts.

★ Does your bowl want to be moved back to center, or repaired? Is there any way your bowl needs to be changed to make it more comfortable for your baby during pregnancy or birth?

★ Once your bowl feels clean and ready, imagine a drain opening in the bottom of your bowl, and let the energy from the Earth and the sky wash everything out of your pelvic bowl.

★ Take a few more breaths, filling your bowl and surrounding your baby with love and gratitude.

www.Genevamontano.com/WisdomFromTheWomb

***

WOMB CONNECTION
PERINEAL MASSAGE

The vagina is perfectly suited for giving birth and does not need to be stretched or changed in any way to allow a baby to be birthed. However, nothing as big as a baby has passed through most vaginas, and it is therefore a very intense feeling.

Becoming accustomed to a feeling of intensity in the vagina can help relaxation occur more easily during birth. Each time this "massage" is performed will feel different for the birthing person. The goal is to learn to relax and breathe, instead of tensing and pulling away, even when there is an intense sensation.

This massage is easiest with a partner. It can be done alone with your own thumbs, if you can reach, or with a clean wand or toy. This is not required, but something some birthing people like to do to prepare the perineum in this way.

General Hints for Partners:

You may use either your index fingers or your thumbs. Sometimes, only one finger or thumb will fit into the vagina at first.

Listen to your partner. It is their body. Be sensitive to what they want you to do. Massage firmly but gently. They will tell you how much pressure to apply

This can be a sensual time. Perhaps some loving touch before beginning will be appreciated. Perhaps it can turn into more intimacy. Sex is good for preparing the body for birth. It keeps the perineal and vaginal muscles strong but flexible and releases helpful hormones.

This does not have to be a sensual time.

Directions:

* Wash your hands.

* Lie back, relax, get comfortable with lots of pillows and support. Sometimes, a bath beforehand helps.

* Put some lubricant on your fingers and on the perineum. A water-based lube or a carrier oil work well.

* Place your fingers gently inside the vagina about one to two inches. Press down at 4:00-5:00 and 7:00-8:00 (the clitoris is 12:00 and the anus is 6:00), until there is pressure and it is beginning to sting and burn.

* Hold the pressure there for about two minutes or until you feel the muscles relax around your fingers or thumbs.

* If desired, gently and slowly sweep your fingers from the sides toward 6:00, pulling forward slightly, simulating the sensation of the baby's head moving down and out. Hold until the muscles relax. Never massage above 3:00 or 9:00.

* Massage any scars from previous births. Evening Primrose oil can be used on those areas. Remember to avoid the urinary opening.

* Massage for about three to four minutes once a day or every other day, starting at 34-36 weeks.

* During this time, visualize baby coming through the birth canal. Tell baby you are ready for this sensation and you welcome the intensity of feeling them come through your body.

* Fears or emotions might come up while you do this. Allow them to arise, and feel them as much as you are willing to. Sit with yourself, your baby, your partner, and see if those fears need to or are ready to be addressed.

* Let your baby be a part of this process. If it feels right, tell baby what you are feeling, what your hopes are for the birth, and take a moment to listen if your baby wants to communicate anything back to you.

www.Genevamontano.com/WisdomFromTheWomb

***

PREPARING YOUR MIND, HEART, AND SPIRIT FOR BIRTH

THIS IS WHERE MOST of us have to do the most work in pregnancy and birth and in life. You, just like your baby, came into this world wanting to learn certain lessons, and your pregnancy and birth will certainly give you an opportunity to learn them. The lessons we struggle with in our day-to-day lives are often the exact same things that come up during birth. It is wonderful we are given so many opportunities to learn the soul's lessons in this lifetime.

Dystocia refers to anytime the birth progress or the baby have become stuck. For example, you may have heard about shoulder dystocia, which is when the baby's head comes out but the shoulders get caught up on the pelvic bones somewhere. Baby is stuck and needs assistance to get the rest of their body out.

The most common kind of dystocia is an emotional or psychological dystocia. This means the birth has stopped or slowed for a psychological or emotional reason. The birthing person is struggling with something, and it subconsciously keeps things from progressing. Your baby will be patient with you during birth, as you figure these things out. However, it might be easier to think about what you need to deal with prior to being in labor.

What are you afraid of? What comes to your mind immediately, when we talk about emotions stopping your labor? Don't think about it too much, just let your first instinct come up. There are any number of things that keep women from feeling safe enough to allow their babies to come out. If you don't feel safe, birth is going to be harder. Period point blank. It is important to deal with these emotions, to give you and your baby the best chance at having the birth you want.

Epigenetics have proven that we also carry the experiences of our ancestors in our DNA. This is a fascinating field that some people might want to learn more about, especially if they feel like they carry a great deal of familial trauma. Epigenetics proves that our experiences change our DNA. The experiences of our ancestors (and this can be our parents and grandparents, as well as those further back) became gene mutations that they passed on to their children and grandchildren.

Our cells and our DNA actually learn from the situations they are exposed to and adapt to their environments. These are permanent changes in the code of our DNA that are inherited by our children and our children's children. So, your ancestor's birth experiences will affect yours and your baby's. What were your mother's pregnancies and births like? What were your grandmother's pregnancies and births like? Ask them. Ask them what your great-grandparents' births were like. You are carrying their stories as you are carrying this baby. We don't realize how much their stories affect us, even when we are not consciously aware of them.

We talk about various diseases running in family lines, but some of them are not actually genetic. Diabetes and cancer, for example, are not necessarily genetic diseases. But if you are told your whole life that everyone in your family gets diabetes or cancer, and your whole family eats a certain way and follows a certain lifestyle, then you are more likely to have diabetes or cancer. Partially from a belief that you will, partially because of the environment you were raised in, and partially because previous family experiences have changed the codes in your DNA. Stories and environment do not have to dictate your health.

The same is true with your birth. What stories have you been told that everyone in your family does or experiences during birth? Is there a history of birth trauma in your family? Has anyone died in childbirth? Are babies born healthy? Have there been a lot of cesarean births? Does everyone birth so fast, they don't make it to the hospital? Start investigating your family stories.

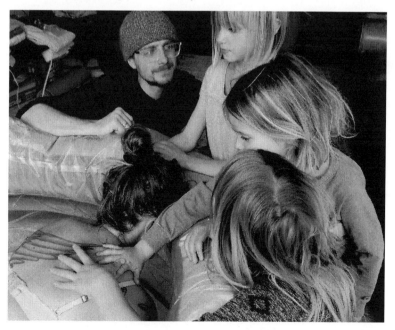

You do not have to accept these family stories as your own, but it is important you acknowledge them, so you can begin to heal them. You and your baby are creating your own story right now. By doing the work to create a different experience for you and your baby, you can bring healing to your ancestral line. You, right now, (yes, little old you!) can heal seven generations back and seven generations forward. This is a concept talked about in the Bible and believed in most spiritual traditions. How amazing is it that you and your baby have the opportunity to heal the wounds of your ancestors and create a new story for those who come after you?

What can your baby tell you about the stories babies have carried in your family? If you feel differences in fetal movement, or if a flood of emotions or hormones come on when certain topics are discussed, this could be a sign that your baby is reacting to these stories.

Do you know that your baby was also inside your mother's womb? Your mother's stories and fears are in your egg cells, because those cells were already in your ovaries while you were inside your mother's body. Your egg cell is half of what became your baby. Your baby was bathed in your mother's fears and stories. How beautiful is it that your baby can both hold and heal your mother?

The other half of what became your baby came from the baby's father. Fears and experiences from the father's side of the family can be passed down just as easily. If one or both parents or you or your baby are from an adoptive or surrogate situation, both the stories from biological families as well as those from adoptive families can be carried down generationally through genetics, environment and story.

From time to time, disasters or other unforeseen

circumstances like the COVID-19 pandemic force people to face the possibility of laboring without a support person. This is something that is foreign to us in our day and age and causes a feeling of panic in many pregnant people. They feel terrified at the idea of facing birth alone. I can't help but think of all the women fifty or more years ago who birthed by themselves, when it was never given a second thought. It was expected that they would go through this experience alone with no one in the room to support them.

It is so interesting that that our expectations can change so much in a few decades. In the 1920s, most women birthed at home, in the 1950s, they birthed alone in a hospital, and both of these were considered normal and right at the time— so much so that people who chose something different were considered to be a little crazy.

But the question this brings up is, if this was the norm a few generations ago, why is it such a big deal for people now? Of course, I believe birthing people should have support! But I wonder why it feels so huge and important now. I have a hunch that the trauma felt by people who birthed alone was stored in their DNA. The memory of it is still living in women of childbearing age today. Maybe this is why the prospect feels so terrifying to the pregnant people who face this situation. They aren't just afraid of the unknown—instead, a part of them actually *remembers* how hard it was.

What was it like when you were born? You might not think you remember your birth, but everything that has ever happened to you is stored somewhere in your memory, in your cells. Just because you can't pull it up in your cognitive memory doesn't mean it's not there. It can be helpful to do a healing journey, to try to remember how you felt when you were in the womb. How you felt when you were being born. These are your original wounds, and you are still dealing with them, trying to heal them today, whether you realize it or not. It can be helpful for your own healing process as well as for your baby's birth, if you do the work to discover what these wounds are.

The truth is your baby will also experience their own wounding during birth and will experience even more of it after they are born. We never want to think we will hurt our babies. But you will. I promise you that you will wound your baby's spirit, and they will spend the rest of their life trying to heal those wounds. It doesn't matter how hard you try or how perfect you think you will be as a parent. Your baby has chosen you to be the inflictor of their wounds.

I believe, if you can embrace this idea early on, you can love yourself and your baby despite this knowledge. You can ask for their forgiveness early and often. You can ask for their forgiveness right now. If you are more than a few weeks pregnant, you have probably already done something you could find a way to feel guilty for. Rather than holding on to this guilt and letting it fester into shame, you could choose to talk to your baby about it, ask for forgiveness, and release it.

You can do the same for your mother. After you remember how you felt in the womb and how you felt during your birth, rather than holding blame, you could choose to forgive your mother for your original wounds and release the blame.

As you think about your parents, you might notice triggers or things that come up over and over again. These are usually clues to the original wounds. Things like feeling your parents don't trust you, even though you are a successful adult at this point; feeling unlovable, feeling afraid you are going to get in trouble or aren't good enough, like you don't belong, or feeling like the world is not a safe place to be. These are some of the more common emotions that babies feel in utero and as infants, as their mothers and caregivers have their own experiences and struggle on their own paths.

If you don't feel ready to forgive your mother or your father, you can start by forgiving yourself for holding onto and repeating patterns that began with your mother and father. This in itself is huge. If you can forgive yourself and start letting go of energy that has been held in your cellular pattern your whole life, your whole life can start to change. This is really big work, and it can help to have a trusted friend or mentor to talk to. Some people like to keep a journal to write down what you are feeling as you feel it.

As you think about yourself as a fetus, you will become more connected to your own baby, and you might start to feel more empathy for yourself, your baby, and your parents.

Ask your baby if they are feeling any of the same ways you felt or if they are holding onto any other emotions. Emotions, images, or memories that come up for you as you talk to your baby might give you clues about what your baby is feeling.

Trust what comes up, even if it seems silly. The worst thing that can happen is you work on healing an emotion that wasn't necessarily from your time as a fetus or from your own baby. Any healing work you do can only benefit your baby and the world.

Your pregnancy, your birth, and your baby are a whole new beginning, a chance to make the world a better place. Take the time to make it count.

Womb Connection
Ho'oponopono

Have you heard of Ho'oponopono? It gained recognition when a Hawaiian therapist used a version of this ancient Hawaiian ritual to cure an entire ward of criminally insane patients, without ever meeting any of them or spending a moment in the same room. Look it up!

The secret to it is that everything you see, everything you hear, every person you meet, you experience in your mind. You are responsible for everything you think and everything that comes to your attention. If you watch the news, everything you hear on the news is your responsibility.

That may sound harsh, but being responsible for it means you are also able to clear it, clean it, and through forgiveness, change it.

There are four simple steps to this method; the order is not that important.

> ➤ Repentance
> ➤ Forgiveness
> ➤ Gratitude
> ➤ Love

* Choose something you are ready to heal within yourself or your family and say you're sorry. You can say it out loud or to yourself. "I'm Sorry." You can add more words about what you are sorry about, if you want, but it's not necessary.

* Then say, "Please forgive me." Say it as many times

as you need to until you really mean it and feel it.

* Now say, "Thank you." Thank your body, your baby, whoever or whatever it was that just offered forgiveness—it doesn't matter who you are thanking. Just keep saying it.

* Lastly, say, "I love you." Say it to everything. Feel the gratitude and love in your heart, and tell everything that you love it. Love is powerful. Simple. Effective.

A great practice to bring into birth and parenting.

www.Genevamontano.com/WisdomFromTheWomb

***

Womb Connection
Journey to your Fetal Self

* Find a quiet place where you can lie down or sit down. Close your eyes, relax, and place one hand on your heart and one hand on your baby.

* Feel your breath. Each time you inhale, see your breath moving in through your nose, down your airway, into your lungs, and landing in your heart.

* See the energy of your heart as a small, bright light, and see that light begin to grow. Notice what this light looks like. What color is your heart's light? Are there any spots on it that do not glow as bright?

* After you feel connected to your heart's light, begin to imagine that heart growing smaller and smaller, until your heart is just a few cells.

* Begin to feel your fetal body take shape around that heart. Feel the amniotic fluid of your mother's womb surrounding you. It sounds like the ocean. Hear your mother's heartbeat.

* Notice how you feel in the womb. Notice what hormonal signals you receive. Notice what you see.

* Don't think; just see if a memory or an emotion comes into your consciousness. Can you remember your birth? The first moments after your birth? How you felt during those first imprinting moments?

* Spend as much time remembering as feels

comfortable to you.

* When you are ready, see your heart grow back to its normal size, and travel back up through your body as you exhale.

* Take three deep breaths, and take a few moments to integrate or journal about anything you experienced.

www.Genevamontano.com/WisdomFromTheWomb

***

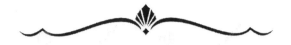

Womb Wisdom: Jaclyn's Story

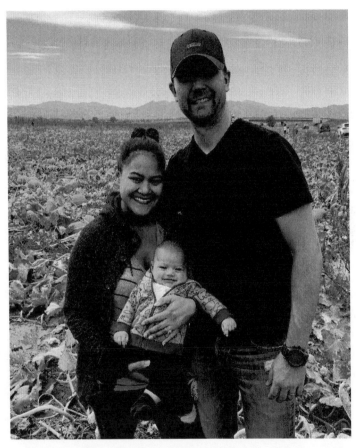

I met Jaclyn when she was six or seven months pregnant. She came to see me for a spirit medicine session.

We cleansed her body and spirit with plants, did some

body and womb healing work, and sat in guided meditation based on the cards she drew out of my Goddess Oracle deck. She drew the Sphinx, who represents challenge, and Inanna, who represents embracing the shadow.

She had a deep connection to the Sphinx and saw herself grow wings as we worked together. I saw her vividly walking with Inanna as she encountered the challenges of the underworld and faced death as a rite of passage.

Jaclyn and I had an instant connection, and I was thrilled she hired me to be her doula. She and her husband, Sean, have such a sweet, loving relationship, and I loved spending time with them and watching the way he supported and pampered her.

I had the honor of leading a small, intimate blessing ceremony for Jaclyn and Sean, where each person present gave both of them a gift. They gave each other gifts, as well. Stones and poetry. They planted seeds with water they had brought home from the mighty Ganges River. We all tied a string around our wrist to keep our thoughts with them and their baby until after the birth.

It was beautiful to attend their birth. All three of us had matching bracelets, and we knew that we had matching intentions to go with them.

Jaclyn's labor started fairly hard and fast, and it was soon getting to be rush hour, so I recommended they head to their birth center sooner rather than later. On arrival, we found that her blood pressure was high, and she had to transfer to a hospital. This meant two long car trips during rush hour while she was having contractions every three to four minutes.

She handled it with beauty and grace, but it was definitely a challenging time for her. She labored beautifully through the night at the hospital. She did everything right. She moved, she rested, she hydrated and nourished her body. She had amazing support from Sean, her best friend, and her mom. But labor was difficult.

In the morning, she decided to get an epidural, so we could all get some rest. She was 9 cm dilated later that morning, and we were all thrilled that we would soon be meeting their sweet baby. Several hours later, she was still 9 cm, and several hours after that, the doctors started giving hints that a cesarean might be needed to get her baby out.

She was 9 cm for a very long time. Jaclyn and Sean were devastated, and my heart was aching so much for them. All her dreams and all the work she had done for a natural childbirth seemed like it was for nothing.

We decided to spend some time in prayer, and I prayed to each of the directions. To the east, I thanked God for new beginnings and asked that this be the perfect new beginning for this family. To the west, I gave gratitude for rest, for the time Jaclyn's body had to gain strength, and for her heart to be strong. We asked their ancestors and all the women who have given birth before us to join us and help her through this birthing time.

To the north, we gave gratitude for everything that grounds us and holds us down, and we asked, no matter what, that Jaclyn and Sean could feel secure in what was happening. We asked all the great Masters who have come before us to guide us and to guide the doctors through this time. To the south, we asked that our fires burn bright and the fire in the baby's heart be seen, that baby show us how it wants to be born. We asked, if there was any way for this baby to be born vaginally, that it be made clear and that Jaclyn could dig deep and be the warrior she is.

During this prayer, Jaclyn reconnected with the Sphinx and felt her wings. She remembered, just before she conceived River, she was at a women's retreat where she had learned about womb dancing. She believed she had danced that baby spirit right into her belly. So there in that bed, with an epidural that had mostly stopped working but still kept her from being able to ambulate, Jaclyn started womb dancing. Each time she rocked her hips, she would have a contraction, and she could feel her baby moving down. She said she could feel her cervix changing.

When the doctors came in to check her one last time, fully prepared to tell her she would need to have her baby surgically, their faces showed their shock and amazement to find that her baby had indeed moved down and her cervix was indeed gone. She was 10 cm dilated and ready to push.

Jaclyn continued dancing her baby down and out until he took his first breath. I again clearly saw Jaclyn walking with Inanna through the underworld, having conquered death, and returning changed.

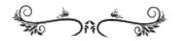

THE PASSAGE
(AKA EVERYTHING YOU EVER NEEDED TO KNOW ABOUT CHILDBIRTH)

SO, YOU'VE DONE THE WORK to prepare your body, mind, and spirit for your birth. The day is approaching. Your baby is growing. You are learning so much about yourself and your baby and how to trust. It is such an exciting time, full of hope and possibility. And although you have no idea what it will hold, other than the final outcome—the baby will come out and you will be changed—if you are like most humans, having a few facts about what you might expect helps break the fear-tension-pain cycle and helps you feel prepared for the birth.

It is important for you to understand birth and your body, so you can feel empowered to speak for yourself and your baby. I want you to know this information, but more importantly, I want you to know, deep in your bones, *that you have always known this information.* You are a powerful, female-bodied human, and giving birth is written in every cell of your body. You don't need this book (or any book) to know how to birth.

Giving birth in the way that feels best to you and your baby is not only your right but also your responsibility. You owe it to your baby, to yourself, and to all birthing people to take back your power by reclaiming this baby's birth as your own. This chapter will help remind you of the normal, natural process. Knowledge is power. This knowledge can't make your birth go any certain way, but it can give power back to you and your baby.

Take the time to feel this information deep inside yourself. Your cells already have this information. Your brain might need to catch up after the cultural indoctrination you have received your whole life that doctors know best, that it is not your job to understand your health, and that birth is strange, painful, and dangerous.

I invite you to remember who you are: A divine creator of life, a child of God, made of the same energy and stardust that created the universe.

Anatomy

Know your anatomy. You have to be the expert on your own body. There is not a doctor in the world who can know your body better than you know it yourself.

Part of how our power as women, as people, as birthers has been taken away was by making other people the experts on our bodies. Our bodies have been colonized. This is why every woman you know, and most men, have experienced someone else acting like their body is fair game. #MeToo. Do you want to stop rape culture? Take ownership of your body.

Do you know where your liver is? Do you know what it does and how? Do you know what foods support your liver? You cannot have responsibility for your health, your birth, or your life if you do not know about your body. The only way to have true autonomy is to have responsibility over yourself. Your care provider is not the expert on your body! You are! And as such, you should know about it.

This book is not going to cover these things in depth. But I feel very strongly that you need to know. Learn about your own body, and teach your babies about their bodies. Learn about how your body can be supported to heal itself. Your body is a miracle. Your baby's body is a miracle.

Be curious about your body in the same way you imagine your baby might be curious, as it starts to notice its own new body. Can you imagine the first time they realize that things appear when they open their eyes? Or when they start hearing their parents' voices for the first time, muffled through water and layers of tissues? Can you imagine what it must be like when they realize they are in control of their hands and feet, that they make them move with their own mind? Your body is just as miraculous. Take the time to learn about it and all of the beautiful, wonderful things it does every moment without you even thinking about it.

Some important things about anatomy for birth:

Your baby is growing inside your uterus. When you are not pregnant, your uterus is about the size of a pear, and in most female bodies, it rests right on top of your bladder, behind your pubic bone. The ovaries sit next to your uterus on either side, and usually one ovary releases an egg each month, which is miraculously caught by a small uterine tube that the egg travels down, hoping it meets a friendly sperm.

When conception occurs, the tail of the sperm becomes the building block of the placenta while the DNA in the head joins with the DNA in your egg. These cells start duplicating, and before you know it, there is a zygote, and the yolk sac is implanting into the wall of your uterus.

This implantation site never changes. Where the placenta starts is where it will stay connected. As the uterus grows and stretches, it can appear as though the implantation site has moved, but it is only the uterus that has grown.

The placenta is attached to the uterus and receives oxygen and nutrients from it, but the baby's blood stays in the placenta and never crosses into the uterus or the mother's bloodstream. Sometimes it is said the female body builds an organ just for pregnancy, but actually your baby is building this organ! Your baby builds a disposable organ from its dad's sperm to support their own life. What a smart baby!

Attached to the placenta is the amniotic sac and the umbilical cord. The amniotic sac has two layers: a maternal side called the chorion, and a fetal side called the amnion. The amniotic sac is filled with amniotic fluid. At the end of pregnancy, there's about a liter of amniotic fluid inside the amniotic sac at any given time. This fluid is swallowed by the baby and then eliminated (urinated) by the baby. Yes, your baby is drinking their own pee. Don't worry; it's sterile. The amniotic fluid is freshly replenished about every three hours. Your body and your baby are continuously producing amniotic fluid. This might explain why you are so thirsty. A liter every three hours!

The umbilical cord has three vessels in most cases: two arteries that carry waste away from the baby and one vein that carries oxygen and nutrients to the baby. If you know your anatomy, you recognize that this is backwards from your adult human anatomy. Fetal circulation bypasses the lungs, which causes their circulatory system to need to be different, almost backwards from ours.

Your uterus is the second strongest muscle in your body. The first is your heart. You don't have to think about your heart beating; you just trust that it will. You also don't have to think about your uterus contracting. Just trust it knows how to do this job.

I'm always amazed that our bodies decided to make the uterus the second strongest muscle. Our hearts work every second or so. But the uterus... How many times in your life do you think you'll use this uterine muscle? Still, your body knows it needs to be strong in order to birth your baby.

Your uterus is made up of layers of muscle that contract in different directions so it can move and turn the baby into an optimal position, push the baby down, and pull the bottom of the uterus, which is called the cervix, up from around the baby's head.

The cervix is a bottleneck part of the uterus that sits inside your vagina. It is the part of your uterus that opens. During pregnancy, it is usually about 4 or 5 cm thick or long, and it is closed. It has about the consistency of your nose. (Go ahead, feel your nose—you know you want to.)

As pregnancy progresses, your cervix will start to thin and soften and will start to feel more like the inside of your cheek. When you go into labor, contractions of your uterine muscle happen rhythmically in order to convince your cervix to get out of the way. The cervix effaces to be about as thin as a piece of paper, and it opens up to the point where a care provider wouldn't be able to feel any of it in your vagina. This is called 100% effaced, or thinned, and 10 cm dilated, or opened.

As this happens, the bulk of the uterine muscle moves from the bottom part, the cervix, to the top part, the fundus, so the uterus can push the baby out. Easy-peasy. This is one of the most amazing functions in human anatomy and the most misunderstood. Your cervix does not just somehow magically open like a zipper. The muscle contracts and moves up to switch from holding your baby in, to pushing your baby out!

Once the cervix is out of the way, the fundus pushes the baby down through the birth canal, which is the vagina. Vaginal tissues are designed to stretch. Just like penile tissues can stretch and grow, so do vaginal tissues. The area between the vagina and the rectum is called the perineum, the "taint" as it's sometimes called.

The urethra is above the vagina, between the clitoris and the vaginal opening or introitus. The clitoris is covered with a layer of tissue called the clitoral hood, which usually connects to the labia minora that protect the urethra and vagina. The labia and the clitoris share similar innervation. Everything mentioned above is covered to some extent by the protective labia majora. The whole package is called the vulva. Everyone's vulvar anatomy is a little bit different, and I encourage you to know your own.

In a non-pregnant person, most of the abdomen is full of intestines. Most of our organs are protected by bones. The pelvis is comprised of two large bones, one on the left and one on the right, that connect to your sacrum, the lower portion of your backbone. The top of the pelvic bones are your hip bones, the bottom are your sitz bones. They connect in the front at the pubic symphysis, what we call the pubic bone.

The bladder and the uterus hide inside the pelvis, and the stomach is tucked under the left ribs, while the liver is tucked under the right ribs. Your kidneys are tucked inside your lower ribs on either side in the back. The lungs, heart, and other organs lie above and between these organs and fill up most of the space inside your ribs.

Everywhere your ribs are, they are protecting your lungs. Think about this when you are breathing. Your lungs should fill up this whole space. Are you breathing deeply enough to bring your lungs all the way to the bottom of your ribs? That is the breath your baby and your body are expecting, in order to get full oxygenation and nourishment and all the chemicals they need in all of their cells.

Your liver does not have its own pump. It relies on the diaphragm to massage it and move all the hormones and toxins and blood through. Are you breathing enough for all the extra work your liver does during pregnancy? It is processing for two, plus all the extra hormones!

In a pregnant person, everything is really squished. The uterus shifts all of the organs that live inside the ribs upward. In the third trimester, your intestines are practically non-existent. Your bladder, too. Give gratitude to your organs that they continue to function, even when their space has been invaded by another life form and they have hardly any room to do their jobs. Your body is amazing.

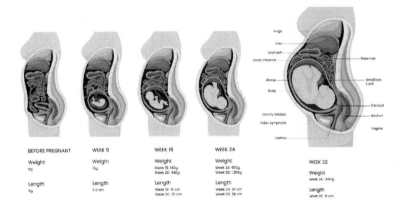

WOMB CONNECTION
EXPLORING YOUR ANATOMY

If you feel comfortable looking at your vulva, it can be really good to know what it looks like before you have a baby. If you are comfortable exploring with your fingers, this can also be beneficial.

* Grab a mirror, sit down, and have a look. Can you identify all the various parts?

* Tell your vulva how beautiful she is. How perfectly made to stretch and birth this baby. From your baby's perspective, your vaginal opening is the light at the end of the tunnel. To your partner, it may be the center of their greatest pleasure. Can you love and appreciate your vulva in the same way your baby and your partner do?

* If this feels awkward or uncomfortable, sit with why. No judgment; just be curious about why it feels that way.

* Try seeing your vulva from your baby's perspective. Imagine your baby's trip through the birth canal, and see if that changes the way you see your anatomy.

www.Genevamontano.com/WisdomFromTheWomb

***

WOMB CONNECTION
GIVING GRATITUDE TO YOUR ORGANS

* Begin by closing your eyes and relaxing your whole body. Notice your breath.

* Each time you inhale, imagine love and light flowing to every cell of your body, every cell of your baby's body. Each time you exhale, allow yourself to grow deeper relaxed.

* Relax your jaw. Swallow your saliva, and feel your throat open and relax. Thank your mouth and throat for the ability to eat and speak.

* Visualize your thymus like a blossoming flower, and smile to it with thanks for strong immunity and healing energy.

* Feel your heart soften and fill with love for your baby. On your exhale, release frustration, impatience, hurt, and revenge from your heart. Let this be a deep exhale. Thank your heart for compassion, kindness, joy, and good circulation.

* Feel your breath filling your lungs. See them soaking up love, joy, and courage as you inhale. Thank your lungs for oxygenating your body. Let them release grief and sadness with each exhale.

* Release anger and resentment from your liver. Thank the liver for its role in assimilation, metabolism, and purification, in kindness and forgiveness.

* Visualize your stomach, pancreas, and spleen, and thank the organs for maintaining healthy digestion, immunity, and blood sugar levels. Thank them for allowing you to enjoy the sweetness of life. Release worry, and replace it with faith and centeredness.

* Come around the backside of your body, and breathe into your kidneys, releasing fear and stress as you fill them with security, wisdom, and calm. Thank them for filtering your blood, balancing water in your body, and giving you more will power and stress resistance.

* Thank your intestines for digesting your food, bringing nourishment to you and your baby, and ask them to continue removing the $#!* you don't need, even though they are getting more and more squished.

* Breathe into your bladder, and thank it for its wisdom in knowing when to hold on and when to let go.

* Fill your womb with a tender loving energy. Your body's place of creation. Give gratitude for all your body has created in this lifetime.

* Connect with your baby, and thank your body for creating such a perfect human inside of you. Thank each of your baby's organs, as well. Spend at least a few breaths here in your womb, sharing space with your baby.

* When you are ready, move down into your genitals, your sexual area, appreciating the pleasure and power it gives you. Thank it for producing hormones

that nourish the mind and body.

✳ As you finish, slowly make your way up your spine, washing the whole body with love flowing from each vertebra through the nervous system, bone marrow, bones, muscles, skin, and hair. Follow your spine all the way up to your brain.

✳ Thank your brain for everything it keeps track of, all the things you are aware and unaware of, all your senses and thoughts. Tell your brain, with gratitude, it is okay to take a break.

✳ Finish your journey behind your eyes, knowing you can always see clearly.

www.Genevamontano.com/WisdomFromTheWomb

***

Hormones

Working along with your organs on a minute but powerful level are your hormones. These powerful chemicals have more effect on your body, birth, and baby than just about anything else.

At the end of pregnancy, you produce the hormonal equivalent of about 100 birth control pills per day. While you are pregnant, you produce the same amount of hormones in one day as a non-pregnant person does in one year.

Most hormone production is taken over by the placenta while you are pregnant. It is working away like a little micro-drug lab right inside your uterus. Is it any wonder you have mood swings or feel different while you are pregnant?

Be kind to yourself, spend more time just being, checking in with yourself and your baby, and lavishing in your goddess state. If you do nothing but lie on your side, meditate, connect to your baby, and eat something delicious and nourishing, you have still done more than an average person in terms of sheer bodily chemical reactions on any given day.

Estrogen is a growth hormone. It makes your boobs grow, your uterus grow, your baby's organs grow, and the levels of other hormones grow (this could be the one that makes you feel crazy). Progesterone supports the pregnancy and helps you stay pregnant. It keeps your uterus from contracting too soon and keeps the baby and placenta safe (also causes hair growth, memory loss). Relaxin also relaxes your uterus, as well as other muscles and connective tissue, so your body will open for the birth (and makes us feel clumsy). Prostaglandins ripen the cervix so it can open for birth (this is found in semen). Prolactin gets your breasts ready to make milk. (It also makes you cry more often and affects mood, immunity, and sex drive).

Oxytocin is my favorite pregnancy hormone. Outside of pregnancy, our bodies make oxytocin anytime we feel really happy and juicy and loved. It is a bonding hormone. It is released when you share a good meal with a loved one, when you get a massage or other touch that makes you feel special and relaxed, and when you have an orgasm. Think about the sweet, tingly, relaxed, and content feeling you have when you experience an oxytocin release in any of these scenarios...

This is the hormone that makes your uterus contract during labor. It's at a level higher than you have ever experienced before in your life. Now, I will never tell anyone that the uterus contracting isn't intense. It is quite possibly the most intense sensation you will ever have in your life. But what if you can reframe this intensity and think of each uterine contraction as a giant surge of oxytocin. With each contraction, you are getting a massive dose of the same thing that gives you orgasmic bliss. Did you know that part of the sensation you feel with an orgasm is actually your uterus contracting?

Oxytocin will make you feel sleepy and wish you could just have a little break to take a nap. It will cause the strongest muscle contractions you have ever felt. But it's just a muscle contraction. And it's just for a minute. When it's over, you could choose to feel the blissful, full-body relaxation love bath that oxytocin wants to provide you. Each giant uterine hug your baby is getting also fills them with oxytocic goodness. You are steeping your baby in love hormones during labor. Take a moment during contractions to check in with your baby—they probably feel pretty good.

Let this make you smile.

Oxytocin is one of the hormones not produced by the placenta; the pituitary gland makes it. When there are catecholamines present—adrenaline, noradrenaline, cortisol, etc.—this signals the pituitary gland to stop producing oxytocin. Catecholamines also send blood to your extremities instead of your uterus.

If you feel stress, your hormones tell your body not to have a baby! Yep, if you are stuck in traffic at 40 weeks and feeling stressed out about being late to an appointment, you are sending a chemical message to your body and your baby's brain that it is not safe to be born. People who decide to work right up until they go into labor often go well past their due dates. The more stressed pregnant people get about their baby not coming, the more certain baby is that they should not come; something is wrong, and they should wait until the danger has passed. This response to hormones is why most people go into labor around bedtime or in the middle of the night, whenever they are feeling the most relaxed and not stressing about things.

Feeling scared during labor does the same thing. A care provider you've never met before putting their hands in your vagina... might trigger some stress hormones! Walking into a hospital you have been to only in times of sadness or panic, a car ride while having three-minute-apart contractions, getting poked with needles under bright lights--any of these things could decrease your oxytocin levels during labor.

Think about this ahead of time. What can you do to keep these distractions at a minimum, in order to keep the oxytocin flowing? How can you and your baby work together to keep stress hormones low and love hormones high? What do you need from your partner or doula? How can you stay focused on your amazing baby instead of situations outside of your control that might be causing stress or fear?

Our hormones are there to protect us and help us have a response when we need to, but we don't have to get stuck in them. We notice and respond to them in the appropriate way and then shift them to a different hormone.

You are teaching your baby, even when they feel stressed, they can shift out of stress and into love quickly and easily.

***

Womb Connection
Shifting Adrenaline to Oxytocin

Adapted from Karen Strange's neonatal resuscitation class

Whatever emotions you feel create a hormonal response in your body. Whatever hormones are in your body then affect your baby. When you feel stressed, you release adrenaline or cortisol, and your baby feels that. They also experience a stress response.

This can often feel like a lot, to a pregnant person, and cause them to feel guilt or shame about all the times they have been stressed out. The beautiful thing about our hormones is that we can shift them.

* When you feel yourself experiencing stress and you know you are releasing a stress hormone, notice it. Acknowledge it.

* Take a breath and talk to your baby. "Baby, this really stressful thing just happened. I want you to know it has nothing to do with you and that you are safe."

* Take another breath. Maybe two or three more breaths. "Baby, I want you to know that I love you. I really, really love you."

When you take a breath and feel the love you have for your baby, your body automatically releases oxytocin. You will feel this, and your baby will feel this. You are not only shifting this hormone for both of you in the moment, you are also teaching your baby that, for the rest of their life, they can also shift their hormones.

***

Signs of Labor

Most pregnant women are looking for signs all the time that they are or are not going into labor, so let's diffuse some myths and review some facts.

- ❖ **Nesting**: Nesting is something that happens throughout pregnancy, where pregnant people want to stay close to home and get things ready for their baby. This is a built-in safety mechanism that starts to get stronger as your baby's birthday approaches. True nesting as a sign of labor is a burst of energy and strong desire to get everything done; it usually happens about twenty-four hours before labor.

  You can't know if any given burst of energy is the one that is announcing labor. So, it's best to keep everything in moderation and never overtire yourself. Your baby does not care if your to-do list is done, if their laundry is folded and organized, or the nursery is painted. They want to sleep on your chest and eat every two hours. They don't care where this takes place or how pretty or clean this place is.

  If you cannot let go or rest until every little thing is perfect, by all means, work on the things you need to. However, talk to your baby about these things. Perhaps they can reassure you that all their needs are met, and as long you have a a safe place for you and baby to bond, a car seat to keep baby safe when being transported by vehicle, some things to keep baby warm, somewhere for them to poop, food to nourish yourself, and a lot of love to give, all is well.

❖ **Lightening**: Babies drop, or engage into the pelvis, sometime in the last month of pregnancy. Sometime in the last month! You could have a baby in your pelvis for a month or for an hour. Not a great sign of imminent labor. Where do you feel your baby? If your appetite gets stronger, you can breathe easier, and you have to pee more than ever, baby may have dropped.

❖ **Losing your mucus plug:** Prostaglandins create mucus in the body, and some of this mucus gets trapped inside the cervix. (The cervix has two openings, one in the vagina, the external os, and one in the uterus, the internal os. The mucus hides between these two openings.) As your cervix starts to ripen, soften, and open a little, the mucus plug falls out. Your baby is still safely tucked away from the world inside the amniotic sac.

There is nothing risky about not having a mucus plug, and your body will continue to produce mucus. You can still take a bath, have sex, go about your normal life. About half of pregnant people notice when they lose their mucus plug; everyone else flushes it down the toilet or some other glamorous thing. Those who do notice it say it looks like a big hunk of mucus. Like a big booger—yellowish with tinges of blood from the capillaries of the cervix. They usually notice it sometime in the last weeks of pregnancy. Yep, somewhere between two weeks and an hour before baby is born.

- ❖ **Show**: Now, bloody show is a better sign of labor, although about a quarter of birthing people do not ever have it. Your cervix has a ton of capillaries, and those capillaries burst as the cervix opens, causing some mild bleeding. This blood is usually mixed with heavy mucus. It increases as labor progresses. It is a sign that your cervix is changing.

  Bloody mucus is a great sign during labor and nothing to worry about. Thank your baby that things are moving along, and keep up the good work. Blood, on the other hand, like blood running down your leg or soaking a pad—this is a warning sign and worth an immediate call to your care provider. Talk to your baby. Are they safe? What do they need from you?

- ❖ **Rupture of membranes**: In the media, it seems like everyone's water breaks as the first sign of labor and then it's a mad rush to the hospital. This, in most cases, is not true. Only about fifteen percent of people will have their water break before contractions begin. When birth is normal and uninterrupted, the water usually breaks at the very end of labor, from the force of strong, regular contractions over a period of time. Some babies are even born in their amniotic sac, and in many cultures, this is seen as a good omen or a sign of a gifted baby.

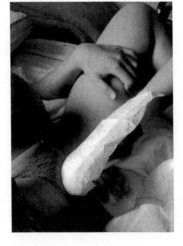

The water acts as a cushion around the baby during labor, helps them move so they can assist in positioning themselves during labor, and offers a small barrier between baby's hard head and your heavily innervated cervix. Often, when the bag breaks first, before labor begins, it is due to the baby being in a non-optimal position and therefore putting pressure on the bag in an unusual way. And sometimes it is due to inadequate nutrition.

Sometimes when the water breaks, it is a pretty big gush, but often it is more of a trickle, especially if strong contractions are not present. For some women, labor will start soon after the water breaks, but for many women, it takes much longer. An entire day or more, sometimes.

It is important to check in with your baby often after your water breaks. Their whole environment just changed! Explain to baby what is happening, how things might feel different. Ask them how they are doing and if they need anything.

Amniotic fluid should not have a strong odor. If it smells like pee, you probably peed; if it smells like your vagina, it's probably discharge; and if it smells bad, there could be an infection. Fluid should be clear. If it looks like pea soup or has chunks of brown or green in it or has large amounts of bright-red blood in it, this can be a sign of distress. (Brown or green is meconium; it's the baby's first bowel movement. When a baby has gestated closer to 42 weeks, they may release their bowels in utero, and this can be normal. When a baby has had an episode of distress, they do the same.) Call your care provider immediately if fluid is not clear.

Once your water breaks, you will continue leaking fluid until the baby is born. If you're not sure if your water broke, put on a pad, and notice if it is continuously getting wet.

Your care provider will want to know when your water breaks. It is good for you to know ahead of time what your care provider's protocols are, if your water breaks before labor begins. This is a common reason for induction.

There is a lot of fear around getting an infection after the water has broken. It is important that you keep up impeccable hygiene after your water breaks and do not put anything into your vagina unless birth is imminent. This means no sex to speed up labor, no checking where your baby is by you or anyone else without some serious thought. Every time something goes in your vagina, it increases the risk of infection. Otherwise, the outward flow of amniotic fluid should usually keep tiny intruders out.

If your water is broken, your care provider might present you with difficult choices about inducing or augmenting labor and other interventions. With every decision you make, you can take a pause, take a breath, and allow your baby to weigh in as well. The connection you have developed with your baby should make this quick and easy. If your baby is telling you something may not be right, you can almost always ask for more time to think about things before you make a decision.

❖ **Contractions**: These are the most reliable signs of labor, as long as they are true labor contractions. Some people have a lot of warm-up contractions, called prodromal labor, and this can be tricky.

True labor contractions always get longer, stronger, and closer together. They are rhythmic, and once they form a pattern, you can almost set a clock to their regularity. They feel most similar to menstrual cramps.

The uterus is a muscle, so it practices contracting to keep itself in shape while you are pregnant (and actually even when you are not pregnant), and these toning contractions are normal. Sometimes, the uterus contracts due to irritability, usually caused by dehydration, mineral deficiencies, or stress. Sometimes, it's from baby moving a lot or a full bladder or just from walking or sex, or it could be there is something else going on with baby.

Always listen and check in with baby, and trust yourself if you are getting the message that something is not right. When you start noticing regular contractions, nourish and hydrate yourself, rest, connect with baby, and if you are having more than four to six contractions per hour, it's worth a call to your care provider.

When true labor starts, nothing you do will change your contractions significantly. It won't matter how much you rest or hydrate or what position or movement you do. Contractions will become longer, stronger, and closer together until baby comes. If the contractions are not getting longer, stronger, and closer together, it could still be warm-ups or very early labor, and it's best to rest and take some time to be with baby.

The thing about signs of labor is, though many people obsess over them, they really are not very reliable. You will know when you are in labor! You might second-guess yourself. It might take a while for you to realize it's labor, but I don't know anyone who, in hindsight, can't look back and say, "Oh yeah, that is the moment my labor started."

Birth is one of the true surprises and unknowns left in life. If you have the privilege of waiting for your baby to start their labor, relish that magic. Trust that your baby knows their birthday. From outside our timeline, they have chosen the moment in time when the stars will align perfectly for their life mission to be accomplished. There's really not anything you can do to change that, and stressing over signs that it may be starting will not make labor come any sooner.

Once baby is born, you might miss the special times when you had baby all to yourself. Spend as much time enjoying these moments as you can. They will be over before you know it.

Labor

Labor is divided into three stages. First stage labor is the thinning and opening of your cervix while the uterine muscle thickens at the top. Second stage is pushing the baby out. Third stage is pushing the placenta out.

Stages of Childbirth

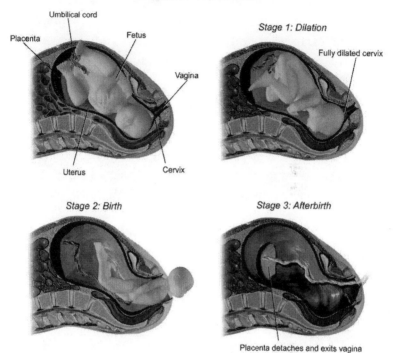

First stage is the longest and is divided into three phases:

1. Early
2. Active
3. Transition

Your baby does not care at all about stages and phases. They honestly mean nothing. No human in history has ever had a textbook labor, and I doubt you will be the first. Even if you do, it's not going to feel in your body like it did reading it in a textbook.

I'm going to tell you my recommendations for labor, and I think they are really solid recommendations. Then I'm going to recommend you throw it all out the window and just listen to your body and your baby. Your body already knows how to give birth, and your baby already knows how it's going to be born.

***

Early labor is defined by relatively irregular, mild (though they might not feel mild to you), or infrequent contractions that are opening your cervix up to 5-6 cm. This is such an amazing, exciting time. It is probably also the most important time in terms of what you, as the birthing person, choose to do. You may be unsure at first if it is really labor or not, but as it becomes clear, it is fun and sometimes nerve-wracking to know that your baby is so close. You will finally get to meet this person you have been waiting for and connecting with every day for nine months. It's going to be magical.

Some parents make the mistake of getting so excited that they think there's something they can do or somewhere they can go that will make this time go more quickly. This is not possible. It just takes as long as it takes. Being at the hospital won't make early labor go faster. Overdoing it in early labor can wear out your body, your uterus, and your baby! For many first-time birthers or when a baby is in a non-optimal position, this part can take a long time. Possibly twenty-four hours or more. (This is an average amount of time. Not a long time.)

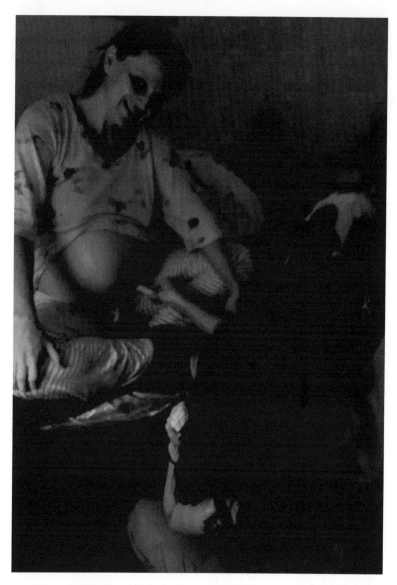

Your body is trying to figure out how to coordinate the three layers of uterine muscles to contract them in such a way that they turn the baby into the optimal position, pull the cervix up and out of the way, and push the baby out.

My recommendation is you sink into this time and rest as much as possible. And when I say rest, what I mean is sleep. If contractions are irregular or are more than five minutes apart, it is a good idea to sleep. Obviously, it will not be the best sleep you have ever gotten in your life. However, any sleep is better than none, and I know it is possible, because I have seen many pregnant people figure it out!

Think about it: if you could predict you would still be in labor in 24 to 48 hours from the excited moments when it starts, what would you have wished you did during the first hours? If labor progresses faster than you anticipate, you can contact me later and tell me you were upset that you tried to get a few extra minutes of rest while you were in labor. (So far, no one has ever been upset about this, even if it became obvious things were moving too fast for them to rest.)

If you cannot sleep, talk to your care provider or your doula, so they can give you ideas of what might be appropriate for you to do. Some care providers recommend a Benadryl, a half glass of wine, a shot of whiskey, Bach Rescue Sleep, sleepy-time tea, CBD, a bath, or anything to help you sleep. If you go to the hospital and are still in early labor, sometimes they send you home with an Ambien or offer you a morphine sleep, if you want or need to stay there. Check in with your baby about all these options, and see what will be the best solution for their birth.

The most common reason women who originally planned a natural childbirth end up deciding they want pain relief is because they are tired, not because they can't handle the pain. Sometimes, a little bit of medicinal help to get rest in early labor can prevent you from more medicine later in labor. Whatever you decide, your number-one priority should be sleep. If you can't sleep, call your care provider.

If your mind is just going and going a hundred miles an hour because you are so excited that your baby is coming and you don't want to miss a moment of it, or you are nervous about how the rest of labor might go, spend some time connecting with your baby. Lean into the trust that your baby is going to guide you and you will know the right time to call your midwife or prepare your birthing area or head to your place of birth. See if there are any remaining fears your baby can help you overcome, so you can rest. Remember that relaxing breaks the fear-tension-pain cycle. You have everything you need to birth this baby. Your body is lining things up, and your baby is just waiting for its birthday. All is well. Find your center, ground with baby, and rest.

It's also very important that you stay nourished and hydrated. Your uterus can become irritable and contract unnecessarily if you are dehydrated. If you start labor in the morning after a good night's sleep and you feel well rested, have a good breakfast. You might feel nauseous due to all the hormones. Find something you can eat anyway! It is important for you to be well nourished, so you and your baby have the best experience possible. You can burn up to 1,000 calories per hour in labor. You and your baby need fuel to do this!

Snack throughout the day, and drink something after each contraction. Have a variety of food and drinks on hand that you love and some that you can tolerate when you don't feel well. Who knows what your baby might want you to eat that day! Think about what your support people might want to eat, as well. This is a big day for them, too, and it's important they take good care of themselves so they can take good care of you.

It's okay to go for a walk while in early labor. Or you can do something you enjoy or a project that keeps your mind occupied. Just remember, it is a myth that you can do any particular movements or positions or push a magic button (otherwise known as acupressure point) on your body that will put you into labor or shift your labor from early labor into active labor.

Sometimes, you will happen upon a position that puts baby in a more optimal position, and this allows your uterus to function more efficiently. Tune into your baby. See what they guide you to do.

Upright positions do tend to use gravity to your benefit, causing the baby's head to put more pressure on your cervix, which sometimes progresses labor in a different way. Walking and squatting or sitting on the toilet might feel nice at times. Doing some juicy stretches to really open up your muscles around your hips while you talk to your baby, encouraging them to find the perfect path through your pelvis, might be a beneficial exercise. You might want to take a bath or have your partner give you a massage. You might practice some of your breathing techniques.

Long labors are often due to non-optimal fetal positions. Your amazing uterus is doing extra work to move baby into the best position. Alternate between resting and trying a variety of positions and techniques that could help move your baby—things like child's pose, lunges, sifting with a long scarf, belly lifting, or ligament releases. You can find demos of these positions on my website:

www.Genevamontano.com/WisdomFromTheWomb.

Spinningbabies.com also has some good suggestions that your partner or doula could help you try. Let your baby guide you on what they need—not every position is going to feel right. Try to give each new technique a chance for at least two to three contractions before you decide if it's right for you and baby. Changing positions can cause a strong contraction that makes you think you don't want to continue there, but the second or third contraction in that position might feel more efficient or comfortable. Baby might tell you it's just what they needed, if you give it a chance.

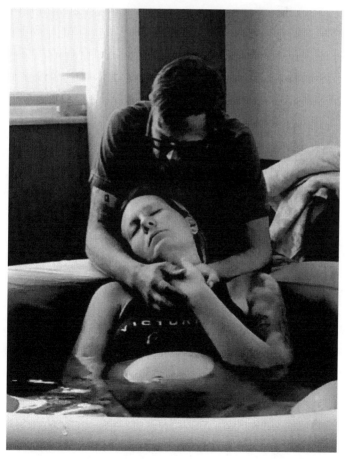

Mostly, in early labor, you should be figuring out how to get more sleep. Find positions that you can rest in, where you can actually sleep in between contractions. Try a heating pad on your back or your lower belly. Put on some birth hypnosis tracks or other affirmations about birth.

This is probably the last time you will sleep without this particular baby near you on the outside for quite some time. It can be a really nice time to connect with yourself and your partner. It's also one of the last times you will be able to connect with baby on the inside. Everything is going to change in a short amount of time. Even if it's a two- to three-day labor, that is a short amount of time, in the grand scheme of things. Relish the magical time you have together during this pregnancy.

Going to your place of birth or calling your doula, midwife, or care provider is always an option, if you need more support. Remember: you and your baby are the experts on this birth. Other people's recommendations are just that: recommendations. Ultimately, you make the decisions. Try to remember to pause before each decision, so that you keep your baby's interests in mind even during the excitement of their birthday. Also remember that your hormones work better when birth is uninterrupted, which means trying to take as few car rides and interacting with as few people as possible.

Early labor is not easy, and how you resource yourself will make a huge difference to the rest of your labor. Let your breath move down into your womb space and surround your baby with your love and energy. Feel the power that your body is creating and just let it be. Ride the waves.

This sounds easy. It is not. But you can do it.

Think about your baby's experience of early labor. Baby

has decided it is time for them to be born, and they have released a hormone that communicates with your brain to start labor. What might it be like for them to start feeling your uterus squeeze them tight? How do they feel, if you are tired or stressed or hungry? What might they need from you to feel safe and loved? How can you connect with your baby during this time?

***

Womb Connection
Early Labor: Letter to your Baby

A fun and simple thing you and/or your partner might try, to keep you connected to baby during early labor, is to write a letter to your baby. You could add simple details like what you both are wearing, what you ate, what the weather is like. You could write about how you both are feeling and what you are hearing from the womb as you know your baby's birth is imminent.

You could ask your partner or doula to add little notes throughout the birthing process as time allows, if you want.

Nothing too serious; it shouldn't be a task, just a sweet little reminder of what this wonderful day looked like. Sometimes people say hilarious things during birth, and it could be fun to keep a log of those things! This could be a sweet gift to yourself or to your baby, in a few years.

(www.Genevamontano.com/WisdomFromTheWomb)

***

Active labor is defined by regular contractions three to five minutes apart, lasting one minute each, that have been happening for at least one hour. (This is the 3-1-1 or 5-1-1 rule that care providers talk about. Usually, first births follow the 3-1-1 rule, and subsequent births follow 5-1-1, but you can ask your care provider about this.)

Care providers consider active labor to be 5-6 cm of dilation with regular contractions. You could be having contractions that feel like active labor before your cervix is dilated this far, and that is okay. Your body is working exactly the way it needs to, in order for your baby to have its own, perfect birth.

There is no math in labor.

Some people dilate from 2 cm to 6 cm in an hour, and some stay at 7 cm for twenty-four hours. There is no way to predict this, and it doesn't have to mean anything about your body or your birth. Each story is different, and you are the expert. Listen to what you and your baby need instead of worrying about a mostly meaningless number. Your dilation tells us very little about the story of your birth.

There is usually a fairly obvious shift when your body has switched from early labor to active labor. I call them speed bumps. Most birthing people have a few speed bumps during their labor, when their body ramps things up and contractions feel way more intense, and they're not sure that they can keep going. These speed bumps are common, and once you get past them, this shift becomes your new normal.

Think about any time you work your muscles. Imagine you are at the gym doing reps of a difficult exercise. There might be a moment when you think you can't do ten more. Your brain tells you that you might be injured or even die if you keep going. This is a speed bump. When you turn your brain off and push yourself through the speed bump, you realize you are fine and you can keep going after that.

Remember: your uterus is just a big muscle and much of labor is mental. Stay tuned in to your primal parts, your intuition and mammalian brain, instead of your thinking brain. Ask your baby to give you the strength you need to push through. You are not doing this alone.

Often the first big speed bump is the transition from early to active labor. Active labor is the time to head to your birthing place, prepare your birthing place, or call your midwife to come to you.

Active labor contractions are intense, and it is often difficult to walk or talk through them. Find your breath. Connect to your baby. Relax around the intense sensations, and let your uterus be powerful. Your shoulders, your bottom, your jaw are loose, and you just melt into whatever is supporting you.

Visualize your cervix pulling up, your uterus tightening and pushing down around your beautiful, safe baby, and let the power flow through your body. Just let it flow. You feel each contraction start, build up slowly to a peak, and then release. The first half of the contraction is building up, and once you feel that intense peak, you know it's almost over. Release it. Breathe. Trust. Let it flow through you. Stay present in your body.

This is the time where you really don't need to think about anything. Let go of thought, and drop into your womb with your baby. You are in your primal, mammalian brain, and your baby is guiding you through the process. Bright lights, talking, strange environments or people, and a lot of questions can bring you out of your hindbrain birthing space and pull you into your thinking brain. Try to avoid these things. Just be with your baby and your breath.

There are no right positions or things to do during active labor. Let your baby guide you. Keep your bladder empty. Sip on drinks, and have bites of food. Try different things, and see what feels best. Many people like sitting on a birthing ball or the toilet. Water is often relaxing. You might like pressure on your hips or sacrum.

A doula can be a great help during this time, to help you trust that you and your baby are doing all the right things. Your partner might need to rest a bit during active labor, so they can be alert after the birth, when you will need to rest.

If you can feel so connected with your baby that you feel like you are one with them, you can tune in to how they feel during this time. They are not afraid. They know what is happening. What feels safe and supportive to your baby? Do those things.

***

WOMB CONNECTION
FIND A MANTRA

When I was in labor with my third baby, I was taken by surprise a little bit. I didn't think she would be coming for another week. So, when I went into labor and did not feel fully prepared, I had to find a way to sink into what was happening in my body and connect with what my baby wanted, which was to be born. I did not want to hold her back or slow down my labor just because I did not feel ready.

I found, if I inhaled and said, "Welcome, baby," then exhaled and said, "I love you baby," my contractions not only felt easier, but I could feel myself opening to her birth. This mantra helped my mind and spirit match where my body and my baby were at.

There are many affirmations and mantras in different languages that might speak to you and your baby. Some people like to put up flags and write mantras on them that they can look at and read and chant during their birthing time. This is beautiful.

My suggestion is that you think about mantras ahead of time, but that the mantra for your birth will be given to you by your baby during your birthing time. See if, during active labor, you can tune in and hear the words your baby is giving to you for their birth. There are no right or wrong words, if you listen authentically.

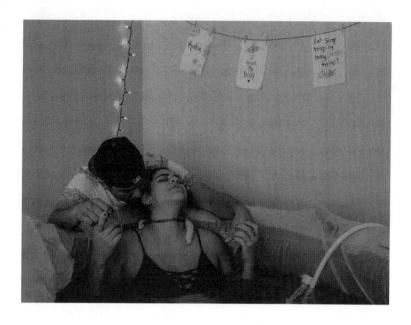

www.Genevamontano.com/WisdomFromTheWomb

***

Transition is usually both the hardest and the shortest part of labor. It is defined by strong, frequent contractions, usually every two to three minutes, lasting sixty to seventy-five seconds or more, that open your cervix from 8 to 10 cm. Remember, 10 cm is not an actual measurement, but the terminology we use when there is no cervix left in the birth canal in front of your baby's head. Transition is the time when your uterus is switching from contracting in order to pull the cervix up, to pushing the baby down and out.

Your body is doing a lot physically and hormonally during this time. Transition is the part of labor that you see in the movies. It can be a big speed bump. You might have hot and cold flashes, you might have mood swings, you might feel nauseous or vomit. You might have no idea what you want, except that whatever is happening is not the right thing.

You don't want to be touched, but you don't want to be left alone. Or you do want to be touched, but no touch feels right. You want to be alone, but you want someone there to reassure you that you are safe. This is all normal, and having your midwife, doula or partner there, someone you trust who can remind you that you are laboring perfectly, that you are safe and your baby is safe, can be important and helpful.

Again, there is no right or perfect thing to do to get through this time. It is intense. As much as you can, bring yourself back to your breath and into your womb, and ignore everything else. A bath or a shower feels like heaven to many people during transition. Sitting on the toilet might be the only place you feel like you can fully release and let go. (It's the only place we give ourselves permission to do this in our daily life!)

The normal emotion of transition is, "I can't do this!" You might cuss, you might cry. Most women ask for some kind of pain relief. This is all normal. This is the part where your old self is dying and you are about to be reborn as a new person. It's not supposed to be easy.

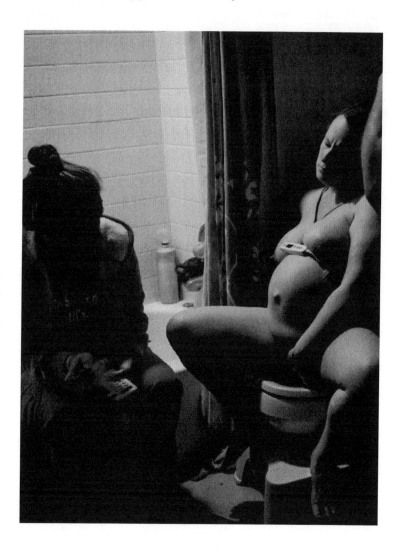

Take one contraction at a time, and connect with baby during each one. Ride each wave with your baby. Feel the power that your body is creating—you are a warrior goddess. Channel that power—the strong contractions are, after all, nothing but your strength. You are doing this. You are almost done. Come back to your baby—they are almost here in your arms. Let baby's wisdom guide and hold you.

Your baby is also working hard during this time to get their head in perfect alignment in your pelvis as they begin their corkscrew moves through the birth canal. Most female pelvises are wider from side to side at the top, and wider front to back at the bottom. Babies' heads are wider front to back and shoulders are wider side to side. In order to maneuver through your pelvis, baby has to make a series of rotations, called the cardinal movements. Baby is twisting and turning, finding the path as your body's strong waves push them down and out.

Babies also have a built-in reflex to kick, or step, when the bottoms of their feet are stimulated. When your baby feels the uterus begin to push down on their feet, baby will kick to help push themselves down and out. When they kick hard, it often stimulates a contraction. Your body and your baby are working in perfect union. Magic. Thank your baby for all they are doing to help this process. The two of you are doing it together, so that you can be united Earth-side soon.

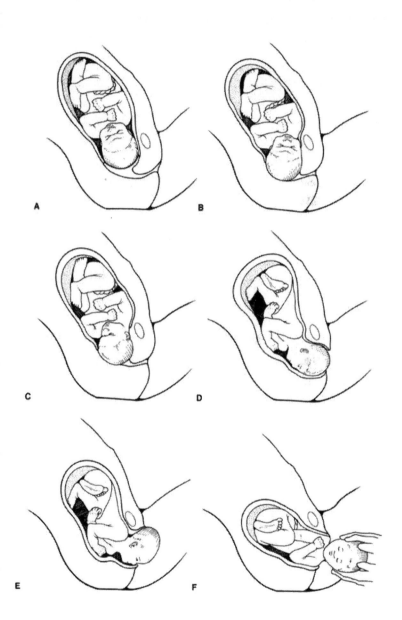

Second Stage begins once the cervix is completely pulled up, and most women who are birthing naturally will feel their bodies begin to push spontaneously. It's not something that generally needs coaching or direction; the body just starts pushing as the baby's head puts pressure on the rectal nerves.

It's a lot like vomiting. You sort of feel for a while like you know you are going to vomit soon… Then, once it starts, there is not much you can do to stop it. It's a reflex. Your body is just doing it whether you want to or not.

This shift into pushing is sometimes another speed bump for birthing people. It takes a different type of fortitude to get on board with what your body is doing during second stage. It is more of an active working with your body, rather than just relaxing around your body while it works. Your body will push, your baby will help, and you will follow their lead.

You don't have to push like you have seen in the movies, but there is some physical exertion in your lower abdomen and pelvic floor, even if you are just "breathing baby down" and not trying to push with all your might. Sometimes thinking about doing a little sit up around baby, or pushing like you are pooping can be helpful.

If you don't have a strong urge to push (this can happen with an epidural or a baby that is not hitting the rectal nerves for some reason), especially if this is your first birth, you might need more direction to figure out how to push effectively. It takes time for your body to coordinate these new sensations and actions in many cases. You will rock baby forward and back, two steps forward one step back until baby makes the turn under your pubic bone. Your tissues and bones will discover how to move and stretch around baby. Baby's skull bones will mold to fit through your bones. First-time birthers often push for one to three hours. It's usually much shorter for subsequent births, but not always.

If you are birthing unmedicated in a hospital, your nurses or care providers may not have much experience with birthing people who do not need direction, so you might be directed to lie on your back, pull your legs back, and push hard during each contraction, even if your body is telling you to try something different. This is a wonderful opportunity for you to connect with baby, find your voice, and speak up for yourself and your baby, to say what you need.

Your baby can be born in many different positions, and your care provider should be able to make the adjustment, if you have chosen a care provider you trust, and you've talked about this ahead of time. Or maybe you can compromise and push in different positions—but once baby is crowning, you will adopt the position your care provider is most comfortable with.

Most women in the U.S., when left undirected, choose a kneeling or hands and knees position for birth. In other countries, where people are more accustomed to squatting, they often squat for birth. A birthing stool or the toilet offer great support and an efficient pushing position. Remember that your baby is also rotating and finding their way during this time, so trying different positions is often helpful. Lying on your back can inhibit the fetal ejection reflex, as well as being anti-gravity, but sometimes a birthing person chooses this position. If this is the case, then trust this is what the baby needs at that moment.

It is miraculous that our babies have a precise path to

follow as they find their way through the labyrinth of the pelvis. It is miraculous that the bones of the female body will shift and move to give the baby the space it needs on its journey. See if you can find a pause of gratitude for these miracles during your pushing time.

It is still important to rest, gather strength, and let your baby do the same, in between contractions. Your uterus is still doing most of the work of pushing baby out, so pushing when you are not having a contraction is not helpful. When your baby is in your birth canal, there is a lot of pressure. Just think about it: a human being is in your vagina. It's a lot. Your brain might tell you to push hard, even between contractions, to get it out.

Again, get out of your head, find a place of trust and connection. Your body and your baby are working together perfectly, and your additional effort won't do much, other than exhaust you.

Some birthing people find this pressure so intense, they either stop pushing or their muscles almost pull baby back up instead of pushing out, in order to avoid the intensity. Sometimes people are surprised at how much pressure they feel in their rectum, and they think that something is wrong, like the baby is going to come out of their butthole. Sometimes, out of fear of pooping, people hold their baby in. (It is literally impossible to push a baby out and hold a poop in at the same time.) Sometimes, during crowning, there is an intense moment where the vaginal opening is stretched to capacity, and you might feel the "ring of fire."

There is no way around the intensity of birth. The only way is through it. Just like life, you have to dig deep and find your way *through* the intensity. Talk to your baby; maybe a different position would help. Maybe your care provider or a loving partner can help physically give you some direction of how and where to push, or a warm compress to offer some relief in between contractions.

This is the final moment of truth for this birth. Where does your strength come from? It's not from your thinking brain or your muscles. Draw strength from your baby, your breath, your support people. Call on the strength of your ancestors and the millions of women who have done this before you and the 250 who are doing it with you this minute. You can do hard things. You are a warrior. Someday in the future, other birthing people will be calling on your strength to help them through their own birthing time. You've got this.

Third Stage

After baby comes, you still have one more stage: the delivery of the placenta. It's anticlimactic, but it's super important. Your uterus will continue to contract, and as it

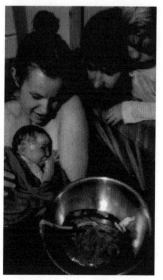

gets smaller, there will be no space for the placenta to remain attached.

Five to twenty minutes after the birth of your baby, you will push one last time and birth your placenta. It's usually about a quarter the size of your baby, and there are no bones in it, so birthing it should be pretty easy, once you convince yourself it is okay to push out just one more thing! Say a little blessing of gratitude to your body and this amazing organ that sustained your baby's life as you officially end this pregnancy.

Phew! Now you are finally done! You can get on with admiring this new human you made and admiring yourself, for being a badass.

WOMB CONNECTION
FINDING YOUR VOICE INTIMACY PLAY

* Sit knee to knee with your partner.

* Set a timer for three minutes, and gaze into each other's eyes. It will feel uncomfortable at first. You might want to look away or laugh. Try to hold each other's gaze.

* After the three minutes is up, move to your bed and set a timer for three minutes or more. Take turns. For three minutes, you will be the giver and your partner will be the receiver, and then you will switch. The partner who is the receiver will tell the other person exactly what they want them to do. The giver should not do anything that is not verbally requested, even if it's something they know the receiver wants. When the timer goes off switch.

Birth is more sexual than many people realize. The sounds that are made, the sensations that are felt, the anatomy involved, the vulnerability needed—they are all very sexual. It is useful to practice finding your voice around sexuality before the birthing time.

How does it feel to be sexual, knowing there is a baby present? Does this change anything for you or your partner?

www.Genevamontano.com/WisdomFromTheWomb

***

Womb Connection
Lion's Breath—Opening the Throat Chakra

* Find a hands-and-knees, tabletop position, and bring your chin to your chest and inhale.

* On your exhale, bring your gaze up to where the wall meets the ceiling. Open your mouth, stick your tongue out, and make whatever noise comes out. It might be a roar, or it might be more of a hiss.

* As you exhale, bring your chin back to your chest and take a few normal breaths here. As you breathe, check in with your body and your baby.

  What can you release? What is no longer serving you that you can let go of before your birth? What are you holding onto that could be negatively impacting your baby that you are ready to be done with?

* When you're ready, take another big inhale, and exhale the lion's breath. Do this until you feel that any pent-up energy inside your womb, heart, or throat has been released. At least three times.

(www.Genevamontano.com/WisdomFromTheWomb)

***

Womb Connection—Rolling the Dice

* Roll Three Dice....

* Add up the total. This is how many hours you are in early labor. What does this look like for you? What will you do? If it starts at 12 a.m.? 12 p.m.? What things do you need to set up, to have this time go as you envision it? Practice with your partner some of the things you might do. Feel into what baby's experience of birth might be like, if it's a high number. What if it's a low number?

* Roll Two Dice...

* Add up the total. This is how many hours you are in active labor and transition, having contractions every two to four minutes. What does this look like for you? What will you do? Where will you be? What tools do you need? Practice with your partner some of the things you might do. Practicing helps get things into your muscle memory, as well as giving baby an opportunity to let you know ahead of time if certain things don't really work for them.

* Roll One Die...

* This is how many hours you are pushing. What does this look like for you? How are you feeling emotionally, physically? How does baby feel with you pushing this long? Babies get tired, too! If your

number is four or higher, this could mean a cesarean birth. What does that look like? What do you need from your support people? Are your feelings around a cesarean birth truly your feelings? Or have they been planted there by the media, stories your friends and family have told, etc.? What does cesarean birth feel like, when you check in with baby?

www.Genevamontano.com/WisdomFromTheWomb

***

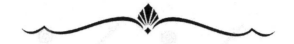

WOMB WISDOM: MARION'S STORY

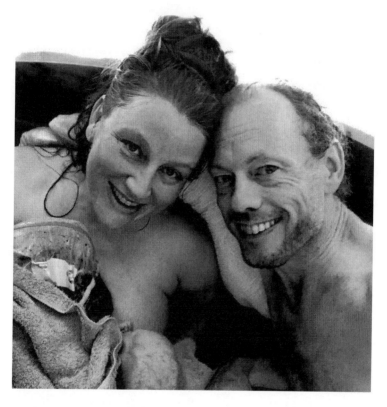

Marion is a forty-two-year-old Bavarian woman. She was pregnant with her first baby when she showed up at one of my birth circles.

She is one of those people who is not afraid to ask any question and comes across as fearless to many American women. She had been told by her OB that she was very high risk due to her age and that her placenta would probably give out toward the end of pregnancy, so she would need to be induced early.

Marion was looking for someone to tell her that her body was not broken just because she was forty-two and just because she had not had a baby before.

Her husband is from Ireland, and the two of them are the sweetest, funniest couple. He travels back and forth to Europe and India fairly often for work, and she is a spiritual junkie like I am, who loves the company of other women. They just want to be loved and told they are not crazy or stupid to think their baby will be safe.

I was a little surprised Marion hired me to be her midwife, only because Jimmy seemed very nervous about the prospect of home birth. He grew up on a farm and had seen many animals birthed, so he knew there were risks involved with birth.

Marion showed up to almost every birth circle and connected with so many other women who were pregnant or had had babies recently. She had that kind of gelling personality that kept all of the other pregnant women wanting to come back and spend more time with one another.

She called her baby the otter. The otter loved yoga, especially Kundalini, but did not like child's pose. The otter had very specific food tastes. Marion, Jimmy and the otter were very connected. Interestingly, Marion also felt it was crucial to develop a relationship with her placenta, to make sure she (the placenta) knew she was loved and important and that she would care for the otter until the birth. The placenta's name was Clara.

I think Marion had a love-hate relationship with my

style of providing prenatal care. Every question she asked me, I asked her right back. What foods are best to eat? Well, what does your baby want to eat? How should I be preparing for labor? You tell me—what do you need to do?

We did yoga together and developed a friendship over the course of her prenatal care. At the end of pregnancy, she confided she was feeling quite nervous that her cervix wouldn't open during labor. She had several friends whose birth experiences included failure to progress, and she started to doubt her own cervix. She saw a body and energy worker through pregnancy, and this body worker told her what her cervix needed was bananas and chocolate!

Marion started having contractions on Wednesday morning. She called me, confident and excited—so excited, I wasn't sure if it was actually labor. I encouraged her to rest and have an easy day, which Marion was always good at.

We spoke later that evening, and I reminded her to get some sleep. In the morning, she called and said she had no idea how a person could fall asleep fifty times in a night, but she did. She had contractions ten minutes apart all night long but still slept between them for eight hours. I have got to tell you, this is the ideal birther! So many pregnant people decide they just can't continue falling asleep in between contractions, but Marion did it for eight hours!

She had breakfast and lunch and continued laboring throughout Thursday. Around 8 p.m., Jimmy called and told me it was time for me to come, that things were getting very intense.

I arrived at Marion's house to see her sitting on the birth ball with lots of energy up in her chest and head, as she was yelling mantras through her contractions. She was doing great, and I knew that, with a little guidance, her energy would come down into her baby and her pelvis. Her contractions were four to five minutes apart, and she was in good spirits, though nervous about what was to come. I asked if I could check her cervix and found she was about 5 cm dilated, just at that first speed bump. We got settled in for whatever was going to show up next.

Marion began to grow quieter and relax into the waves that were bringing her baby to her. She told me that, as soon as I arrived, everything felt right and calm. Together we breathed and centered ourselves as she connected with the otter's peaceful energy.

We used the birth tub, the birth ball, a long scarf; we sat on the toilet, we all took naps. Her contractions would slow down whenever she was relaxed and speed up if she got cold or heard a loud noise. Her cat sat on the edge of the birth tub and supported her through many waves.

She learned she did not have to give her contractions the same amount of energy that she felt coming out of her with each wave. She learned to settle in to the waves and just ride them. She connected with the otter over and over again.

She started to wonder why she deserved the birth of her dreams, when so many others had not been able to have theirs. In the morning, when she started to feel tired and discouraged, she nursed an imaginary otter and cried while she rocked it and nourished it with her breasts. She remembered her warrior poses from yoga class and did them in between contractions.

I watched in awe as I saw Marion change into a mother that day. At one point, while she was sitting on the toilet, I asked her to reach with her finger and see if she could feel her baby's head. She did, and she cried.

Labor was long. I checked her several times, but at the

end, she declined any more exams, because she knew that her cervix just needed to be trusted. She fed it chocolate and bananas and soon felt an urge to push.

She pushed for a long time in the birth tub. We could see the otter's head for quite some time as Marion worked with the otter and her pelvis to try to figure out exactly what energy was needed to bring them into the world.

Jimmy was there, cheering her on. Literally cheering! Invoking the energy of all of their previous family pets. He told me later that he was terrified, but from an outside perspective he was perfectly present and in love with his wife and his baby.

The otter's heart tones started to tell me that they needed to be born sooner than later, so I asked her to get out of the birth tub. Marion had her heart set on a water birth, and I felt terrible asking her to get out, but I knew it was the right thing to do, because baby was telling me so.

My assistant was helping her get out of the tub, and as she lifted her left leg to step out, the otter's head slipped out of her vagina. The otter was born with one of Marion's legs in the water and one out. A creature of both land and water.

Marion said she felt like a goddess rising up out of the water as she birthed. How does it get any better than that?

Marion always knew the otter was safe and healthy. But when Clara was born, her placenta, she cried tears of gratitude. She took pictures and made prints so she could remember how perfect and strong her baby's amazing placenta was. How her body was not broken.

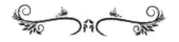

THE DECISIONS
(AKA INFORMED CHOICE)

MAKING DECISIONS ABOUT your birth is such an interesting topic. It is interesting because, in many cases, we think we are making decisions when, really, we are just doing what we are told, what society wants us to do, what our mothers did, or what our friends do, without even thinking about it. If you don't know why you are choosing something, then you aren't really deciding at all.

Have you ever heard the story about the lady who always cut the ends off of her ham before she baked it? While preparing for a big holiday dinner, her daughter asked her why she cut the ends off the ham, and she didn't really know. It was just the way she had been taught by her mother; it was the way it had always been done.

She started to think about it, so she asked her mother why they cut the ends off the ham. Her mother wasn't sure, either, so she asked her mother, the great-grandmother of the girl who originally asked the question.

The great grandmother said, "I cut the ends off the ham because that's the only way it would fit in my pan."

This is the way many decisions are made. We don't actually put any thought into why we are doing things. We just do them because that's the way we were taught. The way they have always been done. Why do we go to hospitals to have babies? Why do we circumcise boys? Why do we get an IV placed? Why do we put hats on babies? Why do we cut the umbilical cord at birth? If you haven't ever thought about these questions, then you cannot make a decision about them.

These things matter to your baby's physical and spiritual health, so get informed enough to make decisions that honor your baby. Medicine is a consumer-driven field, and you, as the consumer, have a responsibility to yourself, to your baby, and to future consumers to question why things are done so we can learn how to have the best outcomes for all.

In some cases, we are led down a path by our care providers to think we are making our own decisions, when we haven't actually been given any choices. You can't actually make a decision when you haven't been given a choice. A choice between chocolate ice cream and chocolate ice cream, even when you love the outcome either way, is not actually a choice.

I chuckle inside a little when I hear birth stories and people say things like, "The hospital was great. They let me have juice and get in the shower." They "let" you do things that keep you healthy, clean, and help you feel good? This is what makes a good experience? Perhaps the bar is a little low here. I chuckle so I don't let out the rage I feel inside that birthing people are made to believe they are being treated well by being "allowed" their basic human rights. (And don't get me started on those situations where people, particularly people of color or those who are seen as "other" aren't even allowed those rights.)

We are given the false impression by some care providers that we have a choice because we are given "informed consent." Informed consent means you are given enough information to feel comfortable consenting to the procedure they are suggesting. When there is informed *consent*, you should also have the option of informed *refusal*. And ideally, you are given informed *choice*, where all the options are laid out with full information, and then you make a choice.

Informed choice is more difficult, because it requires the birthing person to understand a lot more information. Sometimes this is hard during labor. Sometimes it's almost impossible, depending on the situation. However, this is your baby's only birth. It is important you understand your choices, so you can make an informed decision that will be best for your baby and you.

Since I can't cover every topic in depth in this book, I recommend you know where to go for information and that you know how to ask questions. [M]otherboard Birth is a great app with tons of information you can use both prenatally and during labor, to help you with decisions that come up; you can download it. There are several other birth-planning apps available as well, so it should be easy to find one that works for you.

EvidenceBasedBirth.com is an easy-to-understand website that goes in depth into topics you will need to make decisions on. Emily Oster's and Henci Goer's books are full of statistics that might help you make decisions. Use the time you have prenatally to gather information and then, if something comes up during your birth, you can check in with your baby to see where you land with that information. Something could be right for 99% of the population, but if it doesn't feel right to you when you listen to your baby, then you have the right and responsibility to be the 1%!

Sometimes things come up, and we don't have time to fully research them. In that case, it's handy to memorize the BRAIN acronym and ask your care provider good questions.

- B—Benefits: How will this help me and my baby specifically?

- R—Risks: What are complications, cascading effects, or drawbacks to this choice for me and my baby?

- A—Alternatives: What are my other options, and what are the benefits and risks to those options?

- I—Intuition: What does your gut say about this option? (Of course, go back to baby. What does baby say?)

- N—No or Not now: Is this something you could refuse or delay? Or is it urgent that this happen now?

Unless there is a true emergency happening, you should have time to ask your care provider these questions so you can make an informed decision. Ask for some time to think about it alone with your partner or support team after you get full information, if you feel like you need it. Everything comes back to taking your pause, connecting with the baby, and letting them guide.

If a situation is truly an emergency, then hopefully you have chosen a care provider whom you trust to make the best decisions on your behalf, and hopefully they will still ask for consent before proceeding. Your care provider is in control of so much of how your birth goes without your even knowing it. They put up the boundaries around your birth. It is important to remember these boundaries are manmade and not absolute. They are dictated by your care provider's training, insurance policies, peer pressure, and their own personal experiences.

Your care provider has had experiences that shape how they think about you and your baby that have nothing to do with you or your baby. If they were involved in a fetal demise yesterday, you can bet they are going to err on the side of caution today. Erring on the side of caution to you might mean less intervention, but to many care providers, because of their training and the factors previously mentioned, the choice of more intervention often feels safer.

Obstetricians are trained surgeons and medical doctors, so they usually enjoy complicated cases, like things that require surgery and medicine. Normal birth is not where the average OB excels. If something is not normal, you by all means want a doctor around. Doctors are amazing, important members of a care team. But sometimes, it's hard for an OB to sit on their hands and not try to fix something that doesn't need to be fixed.

I readily admit I have a bias, but this is not just my opinion. I have seen doctors walk out of the room because they know, if they stick around, they will want to do something when nothing actually needs to be done. These are great doctors, and I give them so many kudos for knowing when they are needed and when it's okay for them to allow some time and space for the natural process to occur.

I could just be projecting, but I believe when we are honest with ourselves, inside many, if not most, birthing people, there is at least a small part of us that desires an unmedicated, vaginal birth. A piece of us wants to prove that the female body is not broken or strange—that it is powerful and perfectly designed. There is a place in our hearts that wants to believe we can give birth without pain medication or augmentation or surgery. I see this small glimmer of hope in many pregnant people.

However, the glimmer is quickly stolen by conversations with other women or sometimes even with themselves. "Girl, just get the drugs." Or, "You think you're going to be able to do it? Ha! I thought that, too, but I was wrong. I ended up with a C-section. Everyone in our family does, so you might as well just schedule yours, too."

People are talked out of the birth they want because of a fear of failure. The fear of failure, in many people's hearts and minds, is equal to the fear of death. If we fail, we let that failure convince us it means something terrible about us. It reminds us of our original wounds that tell us we are weak, unlovable, unsafe, so why even try? We worry so much about what other people think of us. We don't want them to be proven right, if they tell us we can't succeed at something. It feels safer not to try than it does to try and fail.

Sometimes, we are also afraid to succeed. We start questioning who we are to think we should have a magical, sacred, powerful birth, when so many other people have not been able to. Some people feel almost a sense of shame when they have a beautiful birth. They don't share their stories because they don't want to make other people feel less than adequate that they did not have the birth they hoped for.

As Marianne Williamson said, "Our greatest fear is not that we are inadequate. Our deepest fear is that we are powerful beyond measure. It is our light, not our darkness, that most frightens us. We ask ourselves, 'Who am I to be brilliant, gorgeous, talented, fabulous?' Actually, who are you *not* to be? Your playing small does not serve the world. We were born to make manifest the glory of God that is within us. And as we let our own light shine, we unconsciously give other people permission to do the same."

I implore you, through your birth, to give your baby permission to shine bright. To give your friends and neighbors and the people you meet in the future at the grocery store permission to plan the births they really want. I implore you to give yourself permission to have the birth you want.

Do you want to have an uninterrupted birth? Why not try to make the best decisions possible to make that happen? Even if it feels scary, can you step out of your comfort zone to trust that you can do it—or at least try? If you hear your baby's still, small voice that saying that they want to be born without intervention, trust that they know intimately, from the inside, that your body can give birth and the birthing process works!

I encourage you to honor the baby's voice and not succumb to the fear someone else wants you to have because of their experience. Do you want a scheduled cesarean? Then figure out the best decisions you can make to keep you and your baby safe within the confines of a cesarean birth. Do you want a home birth? Then who cares if your parents or your neighbors think you are crazy? In reality, there are horror stories about every side of every decision you could make. Making a decision based on someone else's stories or thoughts will *never* bring you the peace or joy you seek.

If you know for certain in your heart that you should have pain meds or be induced or have a cesarean, I would never in a million years argue with you. You are the expert on your body and your baby. No matter what anyone else tells you. Your doctor, your mother, your partner, or me. Please do not listen to me about any of this, if your baby is telling you to do something different. You have to do what feels right.

Only you can know what will be best for you and your baby. And hey—you might even change your mind at some point. You get to do that! You will discover during your birthing time that, just like in life, going with the flow makes things easier. Remaining open-minded, open-hearted, and open to your baby's guidance will make the experience easier. You might not get the birth you planned. You might even wish you had made a different decision. (Although I do not recall any birthing people in my community who planned an intervention-free birth, or even a home birth, and who ended up with an epidural or cesarean birth, saying they wished they had never tried.)

But you can be proud that you took back your power and stood for what you believed in. You made a decision based on what your heart and your baby told you was best, and the information you had at the time. This in itself is amazing. A revolution. This is such good practice for parenting. Taking ownership of your power during pregnancy and birth teaches you to take ownership of your power in life.

***

This section is not designed to be a comprehensive guide to all the decisions you might have to make during your birth. But it will give you a starting place to think about some of them. Research tells us that, emotionally, people feel best about their births when they feel safe, when they feel special, and when they feel heard.[10] The physical outcomes are secondary to these things. You have some amount of control over feeling safe, special, and heard by surrounding yourself with people who will listen to you and love you no matter what.

I encourage you to do your own research and talk to your care provider and other trusted friends who have had babies, to see how their experiences of these things went. The options around each of these decisions will vary widely, depending where you decide to birth. Remember that if your care provider's responses do not mesh with your wishes, it could be a sign that you need to make bigger changes. Home birth and free birth are options in almost every community, and the option to go to the hospital as needed is always there. Most community-based midwives offer their clients options, but many things are not mandatory. OBs and hospitals often have more rigid protocols. If something is a requirement with one care provider and not with another, this is a clue that it is something you might want to research more.

Ultimately, every decision should be yours. This means the consequences for each decision are also yours. After you have learned what you need to, let all the information drift away, take some deep breaths, and let your baby lead you through this birth.

Prenatal testing

There are many different types of tests offered in the first trimester, to screen baby for serious genetic anomalies. I encourage you to learn about each of them and then check in with baby before deciding whether or not to do any of them. My general recommendation is that you think about the testing from the endpoint. Meaning, if your baby had a genetic anomaly, would it change the way you want to birth?

Would it change the way you want to prepare for parenting? Would you still have this baby, if you know it is incompatible with life or destined for a more difficult life?

These are deep and difficult questions that do not have a right answer. I believe there are some babies who come into the womb only for a short time, knowing their lessons for this lifetime will only take them a very short time to learn. Some people know, no matter what this baby's genetic makeup or prognosis, they are going to love them and take care of them. Therefore, knowing the health status of the baby prenatally does not have an influence on the kinds of decisions they want to make for their birth experience. They believe whatever care the baby needs after the birth will be handled after the birth. Some people believe in miraculous healing.

Some people never get any testing, never get an ultrasound, and have perfectly healthy babies. Some have many ultrasounds and many tests, and their babies are born with unexpected anomalies. Technology is not always perfect and sometimes offers a false sense of security, and some people are okay with that! Perhaps your baby can communicate their needs to you around testing.

Two of the most common tests people are recommended to have in the U.S. are the glucose tolerance test for gestational diabetes screening and the group B strep testing. In many countries, testing for these two disorders is not done routinely, but in the U.S., it is presented as mandatory by many care providers.

You should always feel you have options in your care and understand why you are receiving any particular advice. You are not required to do anything just because it is your care provider's routine protocol. You have the choice to opt in or out of all care, and your care provider then has the option to determine whether they feel comfortable caring for you, if you decline their recommendations.

Group B strep is bacteria many people carry in their guts. Since it lives in our gut, we poop it out. When it travels out of the rectum, there is a chance some of it can crawl across the perineum and enter the vagina, finding a warm and moist home there. About a third of all women carry GBS in their vagina at any given time. It does not affect the gut or the vagina when a woman carries these bacteria. However, if it enters the respiratory tract of an infant, it can cause a pretty serious infection.

In the U.S., it is routine to test pregnant women around 36 weeks to see if they have group B strep in their vagina. If they do, they are treated with antibiotics during labor, in most cases. Antibiotics, of course, come with their own set of risk factors. The rate of infection for babies whose mothers are highly colonized with group B strep, if they do not receive antibiotics during labor, is about 1 in 200, and if they do receive antibiotics, it is about 1 in 5,000. Not all babies who get a group B strep infection get very ill, but some do. It can be very serious for those few babies. You can do more research about GBS and the testing and treatment and decide for yourself.

The glucose tolerance test is a screening for gestational diabetes. Pregnant people consume 50 grams of glucose, and their blood sugar levels are tested one hour afterward. If their blood sugar is higher than the cutoff, which is 130 for most care providers, then a second test is done with 100 grams of glucose, and blood sugar levels are tested fasting and at intervals after consuming the glucose drink. Some care providers offer alternatives to this test.

Gestational diabetes can be a complicating factor during pregnancy and birth. It can cause babies to grow larger than they normally would, because they are processing sugar in a different way. Sometimes, their chests grow larger, which can complicate birth for some babies. Sometimes, the placenta degrades faster. There are different treatment options for gestational diabetes, and these should be discussed with your doctor or midwife. In many countries, pregnant people are not screened routinely for gestational diabetes but instead are screened only if they have risk factors or are showing symptoms.

Most care providers in the U.S. feel strongly that these tests should be done, but remember, you always have options. Your baby might give you clear direction in one way or the other.

IVs

If you are birthing in a hospital, usually one of the first things that happens when you arrive is the placement of an IV port. It is not always a requirement that you are hooked up to fluids or medicine, but most hospitals are fairly adamant that the port is there. This is done in case of an emergency, so they have a way to give you a blood transfusion quickly.

This might seem reasonable to you, in which case, you will happily receive an IV port and continue with a beautiful birth. Some people though, don't want an IV, have bad experiences with them, or are terrified of needles, and the IV is the most traumatic part of their birth experience. Some people just want to wait until they are closer to the birth before they have the IV placed.

If you think about every other emergency situation, the

medical staff is magically able to place an IV *after* the emergency happens! If you get in a car accident and are taken to the hospital, an IV line will probably be placed while you are still in the ambulance. If the EMTs are unable to get a line in, then the most experienced doctors will be waiting for you on arrival, so they can get you the medical care you need.

There's a good chance, if there was an emergency during your birth, the same thing could happen. In labor and delivery, the staff is often unwilling to wait to see if an emergency happens. Granted, dehydrated laboring people can be a hard stick. But generally, the medical staff is pretty good at their job, and hopefully you can trust them to place an IV in a worst-case scenario.

Sometimes, getting an IV placed and receiving fluids through it gives laboring people a second wind, if they have been laboring a long time or vomiting and have become dehydrated. They are mandatory for things like epidurals, induction, or cesarean births.

There are many varying protocols around IVs, so ask your care provider about theirs. How might an IV affect the rest of your birthing time? Does this affect your baby's experience?

Monitoring

Another thing that happens quickly after arrival at your birth place is your baby's heart rate is monitored. All care providers want to check in with baby during labor in one way or another. This may be done intermittently with a doppler or fetoscope, or at a hospital you may be asked to wear external monitors continuously. The continuous monitors allow care providers to keep track of your baby's heart rate while they are not in the room. Nowadays, doctors can even login from home and see what the monitor shows.

This might seem harmless or even beneficial to some people. But it can be uncomfortable, it can cause fear, and it does sometimes offer a false sense of security. It has also been shown that continuous monitoring increases the rate of cesarean birth unnecessarily. Babies have fluctuations in their heart rates, and this can be normal and does not always require surgery.

It is important to know how baby is doing during labor. We want to know that baby is tolerating the contractions. This can often be assessed with intermittent monitoring. But once a parent has been told their baby might be having fluctuations in their heart rate, they might decide that continuous monitoring is best. Internal monitors that attach to baby's scalp or are placed in between your uterus and the baby's head can give a more accurate reading, if that is needed or desired.

Fetal movement is always the best indicator of fetal well-being. Your baby can tell you they are okay. You are still the expert.

Most manmade tools have failed to lower the instances of infant or maternal morbidity or mortality. Care providers often use these tools to feel safe. Parents may or may not want or need these tools. Having monitors on automatically shifts the focus in the room away from the birthing person and the baby to a machine. Monitors will change the experience, even when a normal birth still happens.

Ideally, you will have options around what fetal monitoring during birth looks like, and your baby can guide the birth!

Hospital gowns

This might seem like a really silly thing to make a decision about. However, if you're hooked up to monitors and an IV and are wearing a hospital gown, you don't really feel like a powerful warrior. You feel like a sick person. You have the option to wear your own clothing. Maybe something comfortable or something that reminds you that you are beautiful and strong. I recommend something that is two pieces, so when baby needs to be monitored, you don't have to expose your bottom half. Some people like something that is easy access for cervical exams, but if you're not planning on a lot of cervical exams, this might be a non-issue.

Cervical exams

Your cervix is checked manually by your care provider or a nurse, to see how far dilated and effaced you are as well as the position and station of your baby. Sometimes, a cervical check can provide much-needed information and help you make a decision about something. For example, if you are considering an epidural, you might want to have a cervical exam. Maybe if you are 9 cm, you will decide you want to continue laboring unmedicated, but if you are 4cm, you will know it is a good idea to go ahead and get it.

Sometimes, your care providers are wondering if your contractions are adequate to change your cervix, and they might recommend further monitoring or augmenting your labor with Pitocin or breaking your water, or a change of venue if you are out of hospital, if your cervix has not changed for a long time.

A cervical exam is no more than a piece of information to help you or your care provider make a decision about your care during the birthing process. You can get one anytime you want, but if you do not want one, it is reasonable for you to request not to have it. Care providers usually like to check your cervix when you or they arrive, to make sure that you are in active labor, before they admit you into their facility or stay at your house. And many of them like to check to make sure your cervix is completely out of the way before you start pushing. In most cases, routine exams that are not being done in order to aid in decision making are unnecessary.

It is up to you to determine if an exam feels helpful or harmful to you and baby. It is your body, and no one should force you to have it examined without your consent.

Inducing labor

Whether or not to wait for your baby to start its own labor is one of the biggest decisions you will have to make as a pregnant person.

It is not recommended to induce labor before 39 weeks for anything that is not a medical reason. Babies born at less than 39 weeks sometimes struggle with their basic reflexes such as breathing and sucking. If your baby determines on its own that it wants to come before 39 weeks, then usually they are ready for this or they know something we do not that makes them safer on the outside than on the inside. Most people giving birth for the first time are pregnant for around 41 weeks. Some midwives think normal healthy pregnancy can last anywhere from 36-44 weeks, but the general medical community considers 37-42 weeks safe.

Some of the more common medical reasons for induction include low amniotic fluid, preeclampsia, intrauterine growth retardation, or a placenta that is degrading. Some common reasons people choose induction that are not considered medical are a big baby, going past your due date, or convenience reasons, like your doctor is going out of town or you are really tired of being pregnant. Sometimes determining whether something is a medical reason or not can be tricky.

I encourage you to check in with your baby often and trust what you hear or feel from them. You can also request a biophysical profile, which is an in-depth ultrasound and non-stress test of the baby's heart rate that can give you more information from which to make a decision.

If you have determined that induction is the best choice for you and your baby, you now have choices to make about how to be induced. Most care providers will check your cervix to help you determine what the best method of induction is. If this is not offered, I recommend you request a cervical exam. A membrane sweep might also be appropriate at this time, which both irritates the uterus and releases hormones and is sometimes a way to get labor going with no additional interventions.

If your cervix is not favorable for induction, this means it has not ripened (softened and thinned and moved forward), and your care provider will want to start the induction with a cervical ripening agent. The most commonly used medicine for this currently is misoprostol (brand name Cytotec). This is an inexpensive drug that can be placed vaginally, inside your cheek, or given orally. There is a small risk of very strong contractions, which could cause a uterine rupture when using this medicine, so it is a good idea to get full information from your doctor and make sure they know your entire medical history. There are other drugs that contain prostaglandins that could be chosen instead of Cytotec, if this feels like a better choice to you.

You also have the option of using a Foley catheter filled with sterile water or saline to create a small balloon inside your uterus that will manually dilate your cervix. This method does not involve you putting any chemicals into your bloodstream, it cannot cause too strong of contractions, it is easily removed, and it dilates your cervix to about three or four centimeters before the balloon falls out.

An induction that requires cervical ripening is usually started in the evening, and you are encouraged to sleep overnight while the medicine ripens your cervix. This is the goal, but when you're in the hospital, the nurses have a responsibility to check on you regularly. Often, people do not get as much sleep as they hope. Some people choose to take an Ambien along with the ripening agent, so they can get better sleep.

When your cervix is ripe, your care provider will probably want to start Pitocin, if your labor has not started on its own. Pitocin is the artificial form of the hormone oxytocin. It is given through the IV and is started off at a very low dose and slowly increased until you are having contractions that mimic active labor, every two to three minutes lasting a minute each. I have been to many beautiful births that started with cervical ripening or included Pitocin. Many women are still able to have a baby without pain relief when they are induced. However, it is definitely more difficult.

When your body produces oxytocin, it also produces endorphins to match the oxytocin levels, so you are in an altered state while you are in labor. You still feel the pain, but you are not as bothered by it, because you are in what we call "labor land." There are no endorphins in the Pitocin drip. This increases the likelihood you will request pain meds.

In a way, Pitocin and an epidural work synergistically in the same way that oxytocin and endorphins do. When you get Pitocin, you might need an epidural, and when you get an epidural, you might need Pitocin to keep your labor going.

When Pitocin is administered, continuous fetal monitoring is required. Artificially induced contractions can become intense for different people at different rates. Some babies do not tolerate them. Your care providers will need to watch the contractions and the baby's heart rate closely to ensure everything is working well. There is some evidence that Pitocin increases the incidence of cesarean birth.[11] It is important to make decisions with your baby's guidance while being mindful of the different twists and turns each decision can lead to.

Another option for induction or augmentation is having your bag of waters broken. If the baby is in an optimal position, this can be a good option for people who are not having their first baby. Usually, with subsequent babies, once your water breaks, it is a sign to your body that you should go into labor. This is not always the case, but it is an option.

Check in with your baby about it, and discuss it with your care provider. If baby is not in an optimal position, the bag of the waters can actually give them more ability to move into a more optimal position. The fluid also acts as a cushion between their head and your cervix. There is always a very small risk of cord prolapse, the cord coming out before the head, when your water breaks, and if this happens, it is one of the true emergency situations, because your baby's oxygen supply is being compromised.

If you choose this option, it's also a good idea to check in with your care provider about their protocols for how long they will let your labor go with your water broken before introducing further measures to get things going. There is a higher chance of infection for you and baby once your water is broken, because the barrier between the baby and the outside world is gone. This chance goes up with every cervical exam or anytime anything is placed into the vagina. If your water is broken, whether artificially or spontaneously, practice impeccable hygiene, do not put anything in your vagina, notice how you are feeling, if you are developing signs of infection, and check in with baby before the procedure and regularly afterwards, because their environment changes greatly with this!

There are other home remedies for starting labor like herbs, acupuncture, homeopathy, nipple stimulation, or castor oil. Some care providers are not a fan of these options, because they can't monitor baby. But every decision is ultimately yours, and if you and your baby feel comfortable with it, you can research these options further. If you are birthing out of the hospital, your midwife certainly has some tricks up her sleeve to get things going.

Pain relief

Most women in the 21st century choose to have some sort of pain relief during labor. If you get to a point where this is the option you would like to take, you have choices! Of course, something like a bath or deep breaths and support from a trusted partner or doula can be its own form of pain relief, as well as things like acupressure, hypnosis, aromatherapy, and position changes. Birthing people who opt to have no pain medications often report that feeling deeply connected to their baby during the process is one of the most powerful ways to manage the intensity of this time. You are never alone while you are birthing.

If these things are no longer working for you, nitrous oxide is an option at many birthing places, both hospitals and birth centers. It is a low dose of nitrous oxide mixed with oxygen that you inhale slowly through a mask you hold onto your face yourself. In my experience, this works as a nice distraction and sometimes takes the edge off for laboring people. I wonder if sitting still and taking focused deep breaths without the medicine would have a similar effect, but I don't have any evidence either way. Even if the nitrous only works as a placebo, some people really like it. If it works for you, great!

The next step up would be pain medications, usually narcotics, administered through an IV. If you are in early labor, you could request a morphine sleep that would help you rest for a few hours. Then you could wake up and continue your labor unmedicated or choose something different, after it wears off.

If you are in active labor, then fentanyl is currently usually the medication of choice. It works fast and takes the edge off of your contractions for about an hour or less. It does not make you numb; you still feel the intensity of your contractions. It just makes you not care about that intensity as much, and it helps you rest and relax in between contractions. This can be a good option if you feel like you just need a short break. You do have to be in bed to take this medication in most cases, and it does get to the baby's bloodstream as well as yours, so it is usually not an option if you are getting close to birthing your baby.

The most commonly used pain medication is an epidural. The epidural is a cocktail of drugs, usually a narcotic, like fentanyl, and a Caine drug, like lidocaine. They are placed into the epidural space outside the dura of your spinal column, in your lower back, beneath where the spinal cord ends. The medication is delivered by a small tube, or catheter, that remains in your back after the needle that inserted the tube is removed. You will receive medication on a regularly timed basis until they remove the catheter or turn the epidural off.

The epidural bathes the nerve endings in this area in medicine and creates the sensation of being numb. You will still feel pressure but hopefully not pain. The goal is that you still have some movement, so you can be active in the pushing process. The epidural should take away enough intensity that you can sleep. There are times when an epidural does not work or does not provide full coverage and it needs to be redosed or re-administered, in order to provide complete relief.

The epidural is usually safe, and the most common complication is an epidural headache, which can be remedied through placing a blood patch on the area of the dura that is leaking fluid. Some people report residual back pain after an epidural.

When an epidural is chosen, it is necessary to continuously monitor the baby's heart rate, either externally or internally, since the connection of physical sensation between you and baby has been altered. Frequent blood pressure checks and IV fluids are also necessary, as a common side effect is a drop in blood pressure. You will be in bed for the duration of labor, so a bladder catheter will need to be placed, and you will need assistance changing positions. Using a peanut ball between your legs or changing positions every thirty minutes to an hour can help ensure baby can still navigate your pelvis.

Even for women who had previously wanted a natural childbirth, sometimes an epidural is a good option to be able to get rest or to relax tense muscles that are preventing a baby from getting into a better position or moving down through tense pelvic floor muscles. Sometimes an epidural can slow labor down. But sometimes it can speed it up, if a person has been struggling and labor has been very intense for a long time. I can't say enough how beneficial rest is during labor for both the baby and the birthing person.

Though pain relief can take away physical sensation, it does not take away fear and sometimes even increases fear or anxiety. Birthing people still need support, even if they have opted for pain relief. For some people, it is more difficult to connect to baby if their physical sensation has been altered with any type of drug.

Sometimes, epidurals do not work correctly and need to be placed more than once. Sometimes, there is a window of pain that it doesn't touch. Use your voice, and let your care providers and your support people know what you and your baby need to feel safe, if something like this happens.

There is nothing inherently good or bad about any pain relief option during your birthing process. It is up to you to determine whether it's the best option for you and your baby at this time. It's best to make these decisions from a space of trust and knowing rather than from a space of pain and fear. Take some deep, connecting breaths as you decide. Your baby will guide you when you remember to pause and listen.

Assisted deliveries

Sometimes people get their babies so close to the outside world but just cannot get them past that last little spot without a bit of assistance. These moments can be highly intense and scary, so, at that time, it is super-important you have chosen a care provider you trust, so you feel confident that, when these decisions are being made, they are made in the best interest of you and your baby.

Most doctors are trained with either forceps or vacuum, and it is recommended that you use whichever one your doctor is trained on. Midwives do not offer forceps or vacuum deliveries, so you would be transferred into the care of an obstetrician, but hopefully your midwife can still be by your side, supporting you and your birthing process.

An OB will not attempt to use vacuum or forceps unless your baby is positioned in such a way that they believe it will be successful. They usually try only to help for a few contractions, and if it doesn't work, then you might be looking at a cesarean birth. Forceps can cause more severe vaginal tears, as well as bruise or cut a baby's face. A vacuum can, on rare occasions, hurt the baby's skull or cause a brain bleed. The decision to have an assisted delivery should not be taken lightly by anyone.

Sometimes, an episiotomy is also necessary. If it is the perineum itself that is keeping the baby from being delivered, and the baby is telling your care provider through their heart tones that they need to be born as soon as possible, then an episiotomy might be a good choice.

Your care provider will cut a small incision in your perineum to allow more space for baby's head. This can be life saving for baby, but also harder for you to heal from. Episiotomies used to be routine when most women were completely drugged for their births and could not assist in pushing, but they're not common now.

None of these things should ever be done without your consent, even when they are emergencies. An assisted delivery might feel traumatic for your baby as well as for you. If any of these options are employed, I recommend taking a moment to talk to your baby and let them know what is going to happen and why (even if they might already know what is coming). Remind them that you love them and they are safe. Remind yourself, too, that you are loved and safe, and that you chose a team you trust. Give yourself permission to feel however you feel about these procedures if they were not a part of your plan.

Cesarean birth

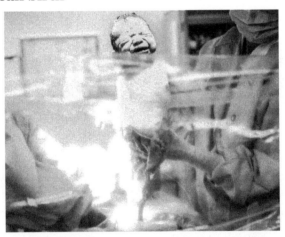

Cesarean births can be planned, unplanned, or emergencies.

If you and your baby determine that a cesarean birth is the best way to go, due to something like a breech birth, a multiple delivery, or a repeat cesarean, you would plan this in advance- a planned cesarean birth.

Some people schedule a date for their cesarean, and others choose to wait until their baby starts labor on its own, so everyone can still get the benefit of the hormones of labor and baby can still pick their birthday. If you are planning a cesarean, this is definitely an option I recommend discussing with your care provider. Remember, ultimately, your doctor can't force you to show up for anything, even for a scheduled cesarean, but you are responsible for your own care and thus for the outcomes of decisions you make. Trust that whatever decision you and your baby come to will be right.

Unplanned cesareans happen when you are hoping for a vaginal birth and, for whatever reason, you are faced with an unexpected surgery. Maybe your cervix doesn't move out of the way completely or baby can't fit through the pelvis in the position they are in, or you develop an infection, or baby is just not a fan of labor. These situations often feel heartbreaking for birthing people, because they feel like it's something they did wrong. In most cases, birthing people have worked very hard to have everything perfect for their baby's entrance into this lifetime. It can feel devastating to work so hard to have what you thought was the perfect birth, and then have things go sideways.

In these types of circumstances, I fully believe the baby knows what is best for them, and they *choose* a cesarean birth. We don't always get to know why things go in a certain way, but I trust that babies, from the other side, can see things we do not, and I trust they know what they are doing.

If this turns out to be your story, I encourage you to spend a lot of time reconnecting with your baby on the outside. Sometimes we learn during the cesarean what the story is—why the baby needed to be born that way. But not always. Sometimes doing a healing ceremony or a rebirthing process or just lying in a tub with baby on your chest in the dark will reveal some answers of why things needed to go the way they did. Healing will begin with you and baby skin to skin. Listen to your baby. Ask them why they needed to be born in a different way than you thought. You may not get an answer immediately, but in time, with patience and love, you will have an understanding.

Emergency births happen quickly, without much time for you to make a decision. In these cases, it is often life-or-death, which can sometimes make it easier for a birthing person to come to terms with its necessity. The most common reason is a baby that is not tolerating labor. Other reasons might be a placental abruption or a cord prolapse. After an emergency birth, it is also important to take time for connection and healing and eventually, hopefully, also gratitude that baby was leading the process.

Cesareans happen in the operating room. These rooms are very cold and sterile. Everyone has to wear masks and protective equipment. There are a lot of strangers in the room who may or may not acknowledge that something big is happening to you.

All of your birth prep techniques will come in handy while you are having surgery. Pull out your affirmations, your mantras, your visualizations. You might be able to listen to music in your earbuds or put some aromatherapy on a piece of gauze near your face on the operating table or in the pocket of your gown. Look into the eyes of your partner.

BREATHE.

Connect with baby. Tell baby what is happening and what they can expect. Tell them they are not going to get squeezed through the pelvis but pulled from the other direction and that they will feel the cold air and the pressure change sooner than later. Let them know they will probably be going to a warmer instead of onto your chest, but that you love them and you will be nearby. Breathe for your baby.

In true emergencies, there are often no support people allowed into the operating room, but if it is a planned or unplanned cesarean, ask if your partner or doula or both can join you. It's great if you can have two support people so one person can stay with you and one can go to the warmer with the baby and talk to them, remind them to breathe, tell them they made it, and snap a couple pictures to show you, while your surgery is being completed.

Getting the baby out is the easy part during the cesarean. It usually takes less than ten minutes. They make a low incision at the bikini line and separate the abdominal muscles then make another incision through the uterine muscle, and baby is out within minutes. Putting your body back together after the surgery takes a little longer. Usually about thirty minutes to an hour.

Some hospitals are starting to offer things in the operating room like a clear drape, delayed cord clamping, vaginal seeding, skin to skin, or they might even allow for you to pull your own baby up onto your chest. Your baby might be able to stay in the room with you or your partner while your surgery is completed. It never hurts to ask. If your hospital doesn't offer these choices, consumer demand is what drives policy change. Even if you do not get to have a family-centered cesarean, when enough people ask for them, the hospital will start offering them, and this will benefit all babies and families and eventually the world.

After the surgery is completed, you will be in a recovery

room for some time. Your baby might be with you, or they might be in the nursery. There are more risks and complications with surgery than with a vaginal birth, so it is important your nurses and care providers keep a close eye on both of you afterward.

Ask lots of questions, or have your support people ask them for you. Check in with your body and your baby often. Make sure you take it easy and let people take care of you. Abdominal surgery is a really big deal for you. Being born surgically is a really big deal for your baby, too. Remember to breathe.

Active Management

It is routine for most hospitals to give you Pitocin through your IV after the baby is born, to make sure your uterus stays firm. After the placenta is born, there is a placenta-sized wound in your uterus that can bleed. The way your body keeps it from bleeding is by contracting. Your uterus itself puts pressure on that wound.

When baby is on your chest, they kick your uterus, which causes it to contract and keeps it firm. If baby is nursing, this releases oxytocin, which will also contract your uterus. Your baby innately helps keep you safe after the birth—how wonderful is that?! Being able to smell your baby also causes your brain to release hormones that help with uterine contraction. (Does baby really need that hat, if they are kept warm skin to skin?)

Some people choose to get Pitocin prophylactically to make sure their uterus contracts and stays firm. Other people prefer to receive Pitocin only if they are bleeding too much. Many care providers recommend the first option—this is called active management—but you do have a choice.

If you are birthing in a birth center or at home with a midwife, you should ask what your midwife's protocols are, and let them know if you have a strong preference about Pitocin one way or another. If you are having an unassisted birth, it might be worthwhile to research herbs that can help with bleeding, placenta medicine, or see if you can obtain an antihemorrhagic drug in case of an emergency.

If you have a very long labor or a very short labor, you are at higher risk for bleeding. Exercising and a diet high in vitamin K and iron can sometimes help prevent excessive bleeding or ill effects from the bleeding.

Erythromycin

It is routine and sometimes state-mandated to put antibiotics in your baby's eyes after the birth, in order to prevent blindness caused by bacteria they come in contact with in the vagina. The most common bacteria that could cause blindness are gonorrhea or chlamydia. You were likely tested for both of these STIs at the beginning of pregnancy.

If you are in a monogamous relationship, you might feel comfortable waiving the antibiotics. If your baby contracted an eye infection from anything other than bacteria in your vagina, you could get antibiotics for their eyes at that point. This medicine does not prevent any other infections or viruses they might get in the future.

Hepatitis B vaccine

This vaccine is given in a series of three doses, and the first is often given at birth. Hepatitis B is a blood-borne pathogen and is transmitted the same way HIV is transmitted. This means it is highly unlikely your baby would contract Hepatitis B in any other way besides vertical transmission. Blood to blood during the birth.

You were probably also tested for Hepatitis B during pregnancy, so if you are monogamous and have not gotten new tattoos or shared needles (It's probably safe to assume you don't plan to let your baby engage in these behaviors!), you have the option to ask your pediatrician about delaying or declining this vaccine if you choose to.

Vitamin K

Vitamin K is produced by bacteria that live in the gut and is one of the main factors in blood clotting. Babies do not produce vitamin K until their gut has been colonized, at about eight days old, so they are at higher risk of bleeding in the first week. There is a very rare disorder called vitamin K deficiency bleeding of the newborn that does not show any outward signs but can be detrimental.

You have the option of a vitamin K injection in your baby's leg, a high dose slowly released over six months. You could also choose to buy oral vitamin K drops and administer them to your baby yourself. Some people trust that Mother Nature or God designs babies perfectly and babies do not need vitamin K.

It is up to you to check in with your baby and then make a decision that feels best to you. EvidenceBasedBirth.com has a nice article on this.

Placenta

All mammals consume their placenta. At least part of this is to prevent predators from smelling the blood and coming to find the baby and the birthing animal in a vulnerable state. However, it is believed there is also benefit to the birthing animal. Research has shown that consuming the placenta can help restore minerals lost during the birthing process as well as regulate hormones.[12]

The placenta takes over hormone production during the pregnancy, so once the placenta is born, no estrogen or progesterone is being produced until the ovaries start making it again sometime later. Some women report feeling less mood swings or less instances of perinatal mood disorders after consuming their placenta, either in a pill form or however else they might choose to consume it.

Some people like to make prints or take pictures of their placenta. Some people like to bury their placenta in their garden or next to a tree or a rose bush, to have a special place that holds the essence of their birth or their baby. Some cultures believe, if you bury the placenta somewhere, it will trick evil spirits and keep them away from the baby. Some people don't want to do anything with their placenta and just want it put in the biohazard trash.

There are some instances at a hospital where the doctor or midwife asks for the placenta to be sent to pathology for research. If this happens and you had your heart set on doing something in particular with your placenta, you can ask your care provider how your care or your baby's care might be different based on what they learn from the placenta, and then make a decision from there about whether or not you want the placenta to be sent to pathology or if you want to refuse that.

The placenta is your baby's special organ that it created to sustain its life. Even if it seems weird, I recommend you at least look at the placenta and thank it for the hard work it did keeping your baby healthy and safe.

Newborn Baths

When your baby is born, it is often covered in vernix and sometimes blood or meconium, as well. It is routine in some hospitals to wash the baby. As with everything, it is your choice.

If you want your baby to be washed, by all means do so. However, it has been shown that the amniotic fluid has a scent similar to the glands around your nipples. Babies will often lick or sniff their hands and then search for something that smells similar, in order to help them find the breast. If breastfeeding is important to you, then waiting until your baby has latched a few times might be beneficial, before you wash the baby.

Baby pee, meconium, and vernix are all sterile, so if you decide not to wash the baby, just know they are not really dirty. At a hospital, as long as your baby has not been washed, they are considered unclean, because they just came through your vagina, and hospital staff is required to wear gloves when they touch your baby. This could actually be an added benefit to your baby.

Delayed cord clamping

When birth happens at a hospital, there are things like insurance and liabilities that must be taken into consideration. As long as the baby is still connected to the placenta, the baby is still considered to be under the care of the obstetrician. Once the cord is cut, then the baby is under the care of a pediatric team.

Cutting the umbilical cord immediately after the birth is a practice that began solely to reduce liability for the delivering obstetrician. There is no medical reason for this practice. It has been studied in the last thirty years to see if it is safe to delay cord clamping, even though throughout prior history no one has ever clamped or cut the umbilical cord of a mammal before the placenta came out. The studies show it is not only safe to keep the umbilical cord attached to the baby, but there are benefits to babies' health for up to six months.[13] We don't know if there are benefits beyond that, because it hasn't been studied yet.

Most of the studies consider delayed cord clamping at intervals of one, three, or five minutes. The longer the cord was intact, the more benefits were seen for the baby.

Most doctors are not trained to deliver a placenta without cutting the umbilical cord, so leaving the cord attached longer poses a problem for them. Midwives generally wait until after the placenta is born to cut the cord. Some people even choose a lotus birth, where they never cut the cord. They just wait for it to fall off on its own, which generally takes about three to five days when it has never been cut. Some people choose a cord-burning ceremony, where the parents intentionally connect with the baby as the link between baby and placenta is slowly severed by flame.

While your baby is inside, fetal blood is continuously circulating between baby and placenta. When the baby is being squeezed out of the birth canal, a lot of their blood gets backed up into the placenta instead of being in their body, due to the intense pressure. If the baby comes out and we immediately cut the cord, baby is not getting all of their own blood from the placenta. It makes sense that babies will be healthier if they have more of their own blood!

Check in with your baby, and see if there is a best time for your baby's health for the cord to be cut. Generally, after the placenta is born, there is no longer a pulse in the umbilical cord, but your baby might still have a specific preference on how long they would like to remain attached to their amazing life-force placenta after the birth. In many cultures the placenta is revered and has spiritual meaning. Maybe being attached to it has special meaning for your baby, as well.

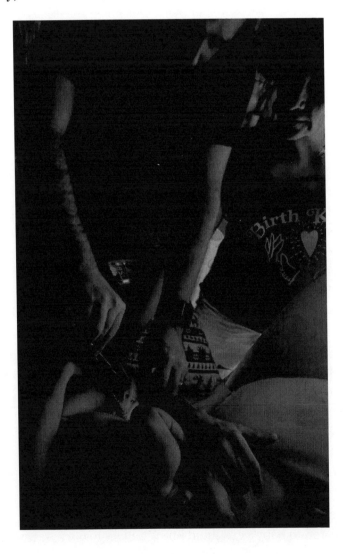

Circumcision

This is a controversial topic, and I will not go into it in-depth here. People feel very strongly about both sides of this argument, and I encourage you to check in with your own baby to see whether they want to have any part of their genitalia removed. This might sound harsh or even somewhat silly to some people, but it is important to really sit with the facts of what happens in this procedure. If you are deciding to circumcise your son, it is an irreversible decision made without your baby's input or consent, and this is something to consider as you make your decision. Please take the time to know *why* you are circumcising and do not take this lightly.

The American Academy of Pediatrics does consider this an elective surgery, and most cultures do not circumcise their boys, unless it is for religious reasons. In fact, in many cultures, it would be seen as genital mutilation, the same way we see female circumcision. In other cultures, it is a very important tradition.

Many times, fathers want their sons to look similar to them, and this is why they choose circumcision. I promise you that your baby's penis is not going to look like his father's. Dad penises look very different than little boy penises, circumcised or not. Circumcision is losing popularity in the United States, and currently about half of the male infants are intact, so locker room jokes about foreskin are soon to be a thing of the past. (About time.)

If you decide to circumcise your baby, I strongly encourage the father or another support person to attend this procedure: To talk to baby and let them know what to expect. To hold his hand and comfort him, when it's over. To listen to baby's cries and know he just had a surgery and it hurts. Babies do feel pain. It is important to remember this and to ensure that a local anesthetic be used for the procedure and to extend compassion and empathy to your baby if he is circumcised.

Feeding your Baby

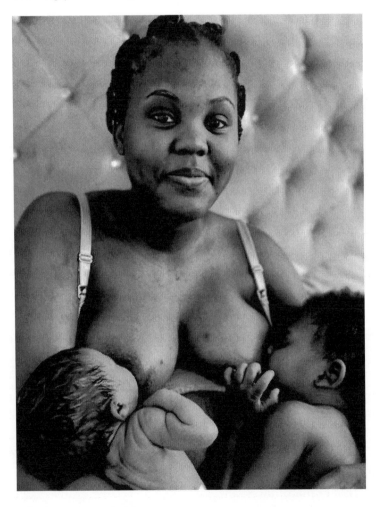

Your baby is born with instincts to survive, so eating will be high on their priority list. Many care providers place an emphasis on feeding your baby in the first hour of life. However, your baby doesn't know how long an hour is; they might need a minute after birth to transition before they eat. You also might need a minute after such a big experience. Some babies will eat immediately after birth, and others will take longer than an hour. When you see cues from the baby, like sucking on their hands or licking their lips, that is a good time to offer their first meal.

Your baby is born with a layer of brown fat that they are planning to use as fuel for the first few days, while the colostrum in the breasts transitions into breast milk. It takes about three days for your milk to come in, give or take. Colostrum is very healthy for newborns, full of antibodies, and nutrient-dense. Whether you are planning on feeding your baby from the breasts long-term or not, colostrum can be a great benefit to your baby in the first days.

Basically, your baby is born anticipating it will be a few days before they get a big meal. Their stomachs are the size of a shooter marble when they are born, so they don't need ounces of milk the first couple days. Some babies also swallow fluids during the birth journey and need to clear those out before they eat again.

In the first few hours, if your baby is not interested in latching, just having them on your chest will stimulate your hormones to start the transition to producing milk instead of colostrum. Keep your baby skin to skin on your chest as much as possible. This is where they feel safe, warm, and are most likely to follow their innate instincts.

Every mammal is born knowing how to eat. Baby kittens find their way to their mother's nipples after they climb over their siblings, suck on a few paws and ears, and eventually latch to the right thing. The mother cat just lies there and lets the baby figure it out. The more you can just relax, generally the better breastfeeding goes.

If you place your baby on your belly, they can use their innate reflexes to kick their feet, crawl to your breast, sniff and lick their hands, then very awkwardly flail around until they find something that smells familiar and that pokes out and stimulates the nerves in their mouth to suck. You can just lie there and let your baby figure it out. You might choose to help your baby, but trust that if you didn't, they would likely figure it out, as long as they have access to a nipple.

Many care providers have been taught to help by latching the baby onto the mother's nipple. You do not need help feeding your baby unless you want it. Most families report more success with breastfeeding when they feel confident doing it themselves rather than having a care provider do it for them. If you want help, there will be help available. Don't be afraid to ask for it, if it's not as easy as I make it sound. Your baby wants to nurse; if you want help to make that happen, there is no shame in that.

If you are breastfeeding and it hurts for more than about thirty seconds after baby latches, something is probably not perfect. Have baby try to latch again or ask for help. If baby is very fussy or refusing to latch, something is not perfect. If you are not seeing many wet or dirty diapers after the first few days, something is not perfect. Ask a lactation counselor to help in those cases. Take a few breaths. Slow down. Go back to that fetal pacing. What is your baby trying to tell you? What is it that isn't working for them? Slow down and listen.

Pumping is sometimes recommended to increase milk supply. Your breasts' milk supply is based on how much is demanded from them. It takes about three days for the breasts to change their supply when the demand is changed. Be patient with your body! It is doing a lot of miraculous things. Creating life, pushing a human through it, turning blood into milk.

Your baby is smart and will take the easiest route possible to get food. It is easier for a baby to drink from a bottle than from the breast. When they breast feed, there is a small amount of food they get right away, but the sucking is what stimulates the food to start flowing, and that sometimes takes a minute or so. With a bottle, there is immediate gratification. If you want your baby to breast feed, waiting for your milk supply to be well established is recommended before offering a bottle.

As a mammal, your baby is probably expecting to be fed from a breast. There are hormonal and immunological benefits to having the baby suck on your nipple, because the baby's saliva communicates with your milk glands to create the unique formula your baby needs. However, there is no judgment or shame in feeding your baby pumped breast milk or formula, if that is what is needed. They just need to eat. Research shows that just two ounces of breastmilk per day, being skin to skin, and suckling at the breast from time to time offers benefits to babies.[14] Do what you can and what works for your family. If breastfeeding is not the right choice for you, talk to your baby, and explain why you are making a different decision. Ask baby what they need to grow and thrive. You will figure this out together.

***

As I mentioned earlier, this is not an extensive list of decisions you might face during your birthing time. However, it is a good place to start. Although I believe that babies already know what their birth looks like, and sometimes we have very little control over this, it is the parents' responsibility to continuously check in and see what baby needs, in order to have the best experience possible. Your care provider has no idea how your baby wants to be born. You are really the only person who has this line of communication and who can give your baby the chance to guide their own birth.

Start today, and every time there is a decision about your care, check in with your baby, and see how they feel about it. Find your voice. Ask questions as things come up, get more information. Then take some breaths, find your way down into your womb, and listen to the wisdom that sits there.

This information is important for partners or other support people to have, as well. In the middle of labor, it might be difficult for the birthing person to make a thinking decision. If a thinking decision is necessary, then it is important that support people understand the birthing person's wishes. It can be very helpful to have a doula or someone else you trust who knows birth, to help you understand your options. However, if it is possible for the birthing person to make a decision without thinking and, instead, simply dropping into her womb and listening to what baby wants, this would likely be the best answer.

If your baby is telling you they want something one particular way and your care providers are saying that thing is not possible, keep asking questions. What sort of compromise can be made? The squeaky wheel gets the grease.

I was at a birth earlier this year, and the baby was taken to the NICU. The dad and I were with him. The dad said he was going to hold the baby, and the nurse said he couldn't because the baby needed some various testing. The dad said that was fine, they could do the various testing while baby was being held on his chest. The nurse insisted he could not hold the baby, and he kindly insisted he could and would. Finally, the nurse left and came back with the charge nurse, who then told this attentive father it was fine for him to hold his baby.

Another family was planning a vaginal breech birth and when we arrived at the hospital, they told her that she would have to have an epidural first. After checking with her body and her baby, they were not interested in this option. The room was growing tense. Luckily, we took a moment to pause, and we were able to find a compromise by suggesting that the epidural be placed, but not dosed.

Listen to your baby, and speak on their behalf. Don't be afraid to speak up for your baby. The worst thing that can happen is the staff will say no, which is usually the answer you started with anyway! Your baby will never have the chance to be born into this life again. Take time to listen and connect with baby now, so that during birth these decisions come clearly and easily.

Remember that your baby has chosen you as their portal and chosen the experience that is going to lead to their highest good and greatest learning for this lifetime. You cannot get this wrong! Lean into the love you have for your baby and the love they have for you in return. Your birth will be perfect.

***

WOMB CONNECTION
CASCADE OF INTERVENTIONS CARD GAME

You will need some index cards for this activity. If you have written a birth plan, you can use it to help you design your cards.

* ✶ On each card, write something you want to happen during your birth or immediate postpartum time. You might have things like vaginal birth, freedom of movement, staying home as long as possible, intermittent fetal monitoring, delayed cord clamping, or baby goes directly onto Mom's chest. You might also have things you don't want. Something like no IV or no artificial nipples, no extra visitors, no vaginal exams.

* ✶ Try to make about twenty cards or more that paint a picture of your ideal birth. Don't think about what-ifs or "well, we would do this if we had to…": Just plan your ideal birth.

* ✶ Now, on the other side of each index card, write the opposite of your wish. So, on the card that says vaginal birth, you would write cesarean birth on the back. On the one that says no artificial nipples, you would write bottle or pacifier. Each card should have two sides: one that depicts your ideal birth, and one that does not.

* ✶ Flip all the cards back to the side that depicts your ideal birth, and put the cards in a 4x5 grid or

whatever grid works for your cards.

* Roll a die or otherwise pick randomly one row to flip over. If you roll a two, flip over all of the cards in the second row.

* Look at the cards, and see if you flipped something over that would require the rest of the scenario to change. For example, if you had a card that originally said no pain meds and you flipped it over, and now you're getting an epidural, you would also need to make sure you have continuous monitoring, laboring in bed, IV fluids, a bladder catheter...

This is the cascade of interventions. The choices you make during birth affect many other aspects of your birth, not just the one isolated thing you are making a decision about. It's important to look further down the road at the big picture.

* Look at the picture the cards are painting now. How would you feel, if this was your birth experience? What could you do to make this still be a positive experience, if it isn't feeling amazing now? What would your baby need, if this is how your birth turned out?

* Roll the dice again and repeat with another row. The goal is to get to a place where you can take a breath, connect with your baby, and know that all is well, no matter how things play out.

* This might not be easy. You might need to take some time meditating on certain aspects of scenarios that strike you as unpleasant. Think about how any scenario could still be positive for you and for your

baby, and whether there are things you need to line up in your life in order for those positive things to happen.

www.Genevamontano.com/WisdomFromTheWomb

***

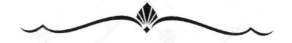

WOMB WISDOM:
ALEX'S STORY

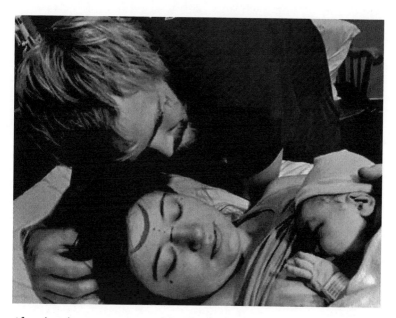

Alex is nineteen years old. She has tattoos on her face and has been traveling for the past several years. Her partner has the word "useless" tattooed over his eyebrow. He is soft-spoken, sweet, and hard-working.

Alex is one of the most informed parents I've ever met. She had done loads of research on home birth and natural parenting. It is interesting to hear her talk about how much more mature she is than any of the other women in her family were when they had babies. Her mom had her when she was sixteen, and her grandma had her mom when she was sixteen. After the baby was born, they were able to get a picture of five generations of her family. How beautiful is that?

Alex had been planning an unassisted birth, but at the last minute she decided she wanted a midwife. She came to me at 36 weeks pregnant. I loved her immediately. She was one of those people whom I both wanted to be friends with and to mother from the moment we met.

She went into labor at 39 weeks, so we did not have as strong of a relationship as I do with many of my clients. But when she said it was time, I believed her. I came to her house and found she was 6 cm dilated. She was handling her labor beautifully at about fifteen hours in.

We got everything set up, and she labored in the birth pool for quite some time. She was singing the song of a birthing person who was very close to pushing out a baby.

As time passed and her song continued, I asked if I could check in with her cervix again. It had not changed. For many more hours we tried toilet sitting, resting, walking, the shower, alone time, intimate partner time, woman to woman time. She got to a point where it seemed like she was struggling to stay focused, and I asked if she wanted to go to the hospital.

She agreed, and we headed in for some pain relief. Alex got an epidural and was able to rest but not for long. She dilated to ten pretty quickly after we arrived, and there was lots of hubbub in the room, because she was a home-birth transfer.

She pushed for a long time with not a lot of progress, which is not uncommon with an exhausted birthing person who has an epidural. The baby started to show signs that it wanted to be born, so the doctors came in to consult with her about a possible cesarean birth.

Alex was very informed about home birth and unmedicated birth but had never looked into decisions that might need to be made at a hospital. She believed with her whole heart she would have the baby at home, and this was a complete switch for her. She asked all the staff to leave the room so we could talk about her options, and Alex decided not to have a cesarean birth. She still believed in herself and said her baby was telling her he wanted be born vaginally. So, she continued to push.

There was a little bit more progress, but the staff really felt like baby needed to come out sooner than later. They came back in again to consult about a forceps delivery. This was right around 7 p.m., which is when shifts change. Alex's sweet and magnetic personality made it so no one wanted to leave her.

She had a nurse and a student nurse from the previous shift who wanted to stay for her birth plus the new nurse and the new student nurse. The hospital midwife who had been working with her for so long did not want to leave her, so she was there, too, along with the new midwife. There were two doctors who were there to perform the forceps delivery. There were a team of NICU nurses standing in the corner, waiting for baby, in case he needed help when he came out. The anesthesiologist came in to increase her pain meds for the forceps delivery. The charge nurse was in the room to help just in case. The amount of energy directed at Alex was insanely overwhelming.

She started to have a panic attack. When I talked to her, she yelled at me, telling me to leave her alone. So many people were staring at her and talking to her and asking her questions, she got to a point where she couldn't even talk.

She just was looking person to person in fear, looking for someone to save her, and screaming that she didn't care how the baby got out. "Just get the baby out!"

She also screamed that she wanted everyone to leave, but everyone just stood there and looked at her. I decided to be the one person who would listen to her, so I stepped away from the bed to the other side of the room.

Alex and her partner looked so vulnerable, surrounded by all those people in white coats and scrubs. I wanted to save them, but I knew there was no way I could, so I stayed in the corner and prayed.

Everyone was yelling at Alex to push, and she was refusing to, so they started talking about a cesarean birth again. One of the midwives grabbed me and asked me to come stand at the head of the bed with Alex again, because she felt I was the only person whom Alex would listen to. And the next moment, Alex looked at me and said, "I'm not doing a cesarean, and I'm not doing forceps. Everyone needs to leave. I'm going to push my baby out."

There was nervous laughter and uncertainty throughout the room, but about half of the people did leave, and Alex started pushing. She said later that, all of a sudden, she heard from her baby that he was coming and she could do this with no help. I don't know if the staff actually believed this was true, but Alex sure did.

The doctors were talking amongst themselves, still deciding whether or not they would honor her wishes and not use any instruments, when all the sudden Alex yelled, "*Did someone just cut me?*"

In a moment when no one was looking, her baby's head just popped out. No assistance, no instruments—she wasn't even pushing. Nothing but the force of Alex's uterus. No one even noticed that the baby had been born until Alex yelled.

Everyone started laughing, and it was such a joyous moment. Amidst the energy, confusion, and worry for this baby and the family, everyone was relieved and in complete shock that the baby basically fell out all by himself, after all of that!

When I asked Alex at a birth circle a few months later if she regretted having tried a home birth, she said no, not at all. In fact, she only wished she would have stayed home longer. She still thinks she could have done it at home, if she would have believed in herself and listened to her baby through the pain a little while longer.

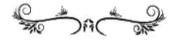

THE RETURN
(AKA YOUR POSTPARTUM TIME)

THE MOMENT YOUR BABY comes out and you see their beautiful, tiny body and hear their cry for the first time is among the most magical moments you will ever experience. You are in an altered state of reality in this moment, where a portal is opened, time stands still, and this new soul enters into our dimension.

There are very few things we get to experience in this lifetime that can so starkly help us remember our spiritual nature and the true miracles of life, breath and spirit. Even the toughest men are often brought to tears by the otherworldly power that envelops the space when their baby arrives. Rarely do we feel so close to the creative powers of God and the energy of the universe.

Take a moment to really feel this. Science still can't explain the intricacies of this moment. You just created life. Be in awe of what you have done, goddess.

This is the shortest chapter and the only one I really want to make sure you fully remember and understand. This information is the most important part of this book. Read it twice, know it, believe it. It will change your life, change your baby's life, and change the world.

Some traditions teach that the first six minutes of a baby's life are when they receive the first imprints for their life to come. What does your baby need during this time?

Think about the experience they just had. They came from an environment where they were surrounded by water and they did not have to breathe to get oxygen. It was warm and dark. They heard your heartbeat and the tides of your bodily fluids constantly. Then, they get squeezed and pushed, and all of the sudden, their world changes.

Babies don't usually take their first breath until they feel the pressure and temperature change of hitting the air. Once they take their first breath, the lungs inflate for the first time, and fluid is pushed out of them as the heart starts pumping blood to them to pick up oxygen that will be transmitted to every cell of the body. Baby is making a lot of shifts in that tiny body! Not to mention the intensity of experiencing a new world in a new body for the first time.

How can we ease this transition for the baby? A warm, dark room, soft voices, tender touches, a familiar heartbeat—all these things could help. If everyone in the room could pause and take a breath, we could be great examples for baby on how to breathe during this transition!

Instead, the standard of care in many places is bright lights, rough stimulation, loud voices, immediately cutting the umbilical oxygen source, shoving a suction device into their mouth and nose, while everyone in the room holds their breath in fear because they are terrified that the baby won't breathe! If only one person at each birth made it a point to treat the baby like a human, communicate with them, be gentle with them, listen to their body language, their cries, and their cues, in the first six minutes of life, if only one person would pause to respect their wisdom, I wonder how things would shift for the rest of their lifetime. Will you do that for your baby? Depending on where the baby is born and what the birth looks like, you as the birthing person might not be able to. Can you make sure someone does?

If babies could be born into a more peaceful, less threatening environment, our whole world could change. If babies were welcomed with love and tenderness instead of fear and harshness, I think we would see a different breed of adults.

***

Okay, so you pushed out a baby and a placenta and the baby is breathing and all is beautiful. You did it! You made the perfect baby. How miraculous are their toes and the tiny dimples on their knuckles, the cute little squeaks they make, and the way they look like birds when they are ready to eat? Your baby is so amazing. It is so easy to fall in love with them and forget about the incredible experience you just had of growing them inside your body and birthing them, giving them the life they have chosen. What a gift. It is also easy to forget what your body has done in order to give them this gift.

For nine months, your baby moved all of your insides out of the way to make room so they could grow. They took all the nutrients they needed from you for their health. They kicked you while you were trying to sleep, and they made you think about things in a way you never have before. Your mind may never have been so busy. Your body was opened up in one way or another to allow them to come out. At the same time, your heart and your spirit also cracked open.

In our culture we forget how important it is to be still and allow our bodies to heal. Instead of honoring our bodies, we seem to honor the women who dishonor their bodies: the women who are running marathons several weeks postpartum or who never miss a beat, who are up caring for their other children and their household almost immediately after the baby comes instead of receiving help and support.

I hope that you will remember you are a goddess. Every god and goddess takes a rest. The seventh day, the Sabbath. You worked hard for nine months. Now is your time to recuperate so you can be a fit and healthy parent for the rest of your life.

Think about this from your organs' perspective. They were squished and shoved, either up into your thoracic cavity or down toward your vagina. Your intestines, I'm not exactly sure where they went, but if you saw the pictures of your pregnant anatomy then you know they were basically non-existent. Your liver, your stomach, your lungs— everything was shifted up. Your bladder, your rectum, and your pelvic diaphragm supported an amazing amount of pressure from the weight of your baby. Your uterus stretched from the size of a pear to the size of a watermelon.

Now, the baby and the placenta have come out, and your organs have to figure out where they live again. If you spend a lot of time upright with gravity pulling downward, especially if you are holding or lifting things heavier than your baby, there's a lot of downward pressure. Where do you think your organs will go? Your pelvic floor, and the ligaments holding your uterus in place, whether you had a vaginal birth or not, have been compromised. All the extra weight of your baby for nine months, plus the stretching from your baby coming through them, weakens these muscles. If they don't have time to strengthen themselves again, all the organs that are shifting downward have the opportunity to prolapse.

That's right, folks. Your bladder, your rectum, your uterus can fall out of or into your vagina, if you do too much after the birth. Maybe not immediately; sometimes it takes years or decades of dysfunction and incontinence before a prolapse. But if the pelvic floor doesn't get to rest and heal, you could be at risk of prolapse for the rest of your life. Take a look at an ad for incontinence products—they are being marketed to women in their forties. Otherwise healthy, vibrant women suffer from pelvic floor dysfunction because they were not encouraged to heal after they gave birth.

Remember all the ligaments that were stretched and causing back and hip pain during pregnancy? Those ligaments now have to heal and go back to their normal state. It takes about twice as long for ligaments to heal as it does bones.

During pregnancy, the rectus abdominis, the six-pack muscles, stretch away from one another. The linea alba holds them together. If this linea alba gets stretched too much or damaged, then it can have a hard time pulling these muscles back together after the birth. It is important to give the linea alba time to heal. When it remains stretched or strained, it can cause back problems, digestive issues, a belly pooch, and general weakness and discomfort that seems to be a mystery to much of the medical community.

Your baby is expecting to be the center of your world for a period of time after the birth—at least the first forty days, but really the first nine months. They are expecting to eat whenever they want, be cuddled close to your body, and have your undivided attention. Your body is expecting this, too. As with most things in nature—the system works perfectly when we allow it to. As your body has time to heal, your baby has time to grow and you both emerge from this time together feeling strong and connected.

Every written and oral history we have reports giving women time to heal after they gave birth. Six weeks, forty days, forty-two days. Sometimes longer. The Bible, Native North and South American traditions, Indian Ayurvedic traditions, Moroccans, African peoples, Island peoples, Europeans and Asians... No matter where you look, women have always been cared for after their births. They were honored spiritually, their stories were heard, and they were kept warm and fed nourishing foods.

I have worked with families from Nigeria whose mothers honor the postpartum traditions. They move in with their daughters for months and cook specific foods that only new mothers are allowed to eat and massage them daily with a special turmeric paste. Women in Nepal to this day leave the hospital and go to their mother-in-law's house to recover. There they receive a full-body oil massage every day and the best foods the family has to offer.

It's the same all over the planet. Women were expected to do nothing other than rest and take care of their babies. Their communities supported them with the best, nutrient-dense foods and round-the-clock love and nurturing, so they could heal and give their babies and themselves the best chance at surviving and thriving. Allow yourself to receive this gift from your community, as well.

This is a great opportunity for you to learn to say "yes" when people offer their support. Everyone who loves you will ask you if you need something. Say yes. Let people bring you food, let them walk your dog or fold your laundry, let them come rub your feet or hold the baby while you shower.

Remember that it is your job to heal and get to know this new being. Everyone else can take care of the other work. The other work is not your job until you have finished the job of healing. Allow your community to take care of you, your household, and your family so that you can focus on your baby. Even if you have the easiest birth in the history of mankind, your body just did something amazing, and it deserves the chance to heal. Normal blood loss at a birth is up to two cups. You will continue to bleed for three to six weeks after the birth, because you have a placenta-sized wound in your uterus. You need to rebuild your blood and give your uterus time to heal, so you don't lose even more blood.

You expend a lot of energy, your life force, your prana, your qi, during the birthing time. This has to be replenished for your wellbeing. Lying down out of gravity, staying warm, and consuming a lot of warming foods help your body and your uterus heal to the best of their ability, so you have what it takes to chase and care for your baby when the healing time is over. Not to mention potentially having more babies, taking care of other children, and all the other amazing things you are creating in this lifetime.

Your body requires 500 more calories per day while breastfeeding than it does while you are pregnant. Every time you feed your baby, think about hydrating and nourishing yourself.

You are not going to get eight hours of sleep, so it is important to learn how to sleep when the baby sleeps. Many people say they don't know how to nap. This is the time to learn! Let your baby teach you. Lie down with them next to your chest, all blankets and bedding away from their face, and let their gentle breathing and soft, sweet noises lull you.

When your baby is asleep, just rest. There is nothing that cannot wait. Your laundry and your emails will still be there.

If you are still bleeding, you have not healed. Even if your bleeding has tapered down, if you do too much, the scab that has formed inside your uterus can fall off, and you will start bleeding again. One week after the last time you notice bleeding is when your uterus has healed. If you feel like the rest of your body is still catching up, please listen and respect your body's needs.

In the first six weeks, exercise is not recommended. Stretching and loving movement in a horizontal or side-lying position, walking to the bathroom or to go sit in the sunshine, or gentle yoga to keep your spine flexible should be enough. However, strengthening your pelvic floor through mindful, diaphragmatic breathing will be beneficial. I recommend breathing into your pelvic floor diaphragm for ten minutes, twice a day. Contract everything up and in as you exhale, and relax everything as you inhale. This is the way your body naturally works—your lungs fill up and everything else shifts down so your pelvic floor relaxes, your lungs empty and everything else shifts up so your pelvic floor contracts up and in (diaphragmatic breathing)—you are just working naturally with your breath.

Listen to your body, and if it feels beneficial, try doing some light stretching while your body is out of gravity, things like legs up the wall or heart openers and pelvic tilts on your bed. Lay your baby on your chest, skin-to-skin, heart-to-heart, place the soles of your feet together, and open your hips (after your perineum has healed!). Open your arms, palms wide, and breathe. Feel your baby's love for you. What does your body need? What can you receive in this moment?

Remember that your baby is expecting to have this time with you. Just with you. Not with you and many visitors every day. Not with you and all the other Target customers. Your baby is imprinting everything it sees and experiences in these first weeks. As much as possible, try to gift your baby your undivided time and attention in these early times. This is what their DNA has instructed them to expect and all they really want or need from you.

There are some great books that can give you more details of how to honor yourself and your baby during the postpartum period. *The Fourth Trimester* and *The First 40 Days* are two of my favorites. We spend a lot of time preparing for the birth, and we forget that, though the birth may be the pinnacle or the abyss of the hero's birth journey, the postpartum time is still part of the journey. It's the return back to ordinary reality. And it is important.

A big piece of this return journey is the mental, spiritual, and emotional state people find themselves in. A large portion of American women struggle with these. Perinatal mood disorders are the number-one leading complication associated with pregnancy and birth. You are more likely to struggle during your postpartum time than you are to have preeclampsia, gestational diabetes, or any other disorder of pregnancy. Postpartum depression is not the only perinatal mood disorder. In fact, postpartum anxiety is more common. And we don't talk about it. We don't normalize how difficult it is to care for a new human. We make parents feel ashamed to admit that they are struggling.

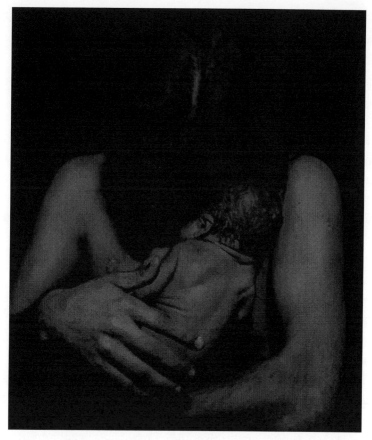

Our society paints this perfect picture of life with a newborn, where the house and the parents and the schedule look exactly the same—just now there is a sweet, cooing, baby inserted into the perfect picture. Let me ensure you that this is impossible. You cannot go through birth, have your bones rearranged, be a portal for a cosmic being, and just get back to regular life the next day.

You have been changed on a cellular level.
Your spirit will never be the same as it was before
you gave birth.
Give yourself some time to integrate the new you.

I believe, if we could take it slower and not try to get back to normal life so quickly, anxiety and depression would automatically lower. If we truly honored our bodies and spirits for the miraculous work that bringing a child into the world is, we would not feel so low. The reason we feel like things aren't right after birth is because they are not! Nothing is right about a woman being alone, whether literally or figuratively, and expected to get back to normal when everything about her feels different. Her heart and her perineum are raw. She is leaking fluids from her breasts, her vagina, and her eyes. Her back and her brain ache from the demands of a new baby.

The things we know that can help prevent perinatal mood disorders are a good diet, adequate hydration, enough support, breastfeeding, and sunshine.[15] I believe, if it was studied, a true connection to your baby would be added to this list.

Not everyone feels an immediate sense of love or adoration for this new little person. They did after all, cause you quite a bit of discomfort physically and emotionally. Tune into your baby and allow them to communicate with you. Just look at them, listen with your heart and your gut. I trust they can help you understand what you are feeling, whether it is through an instant bond or one that develops over time.

Breathing and connecting with your baby postpartum

can help. Sit with them, and look into their eyes. Let them tell you their story with their cries, listen to your baby! Instead of just nursing them, putting them down, and wondering what you are doing wrong when they cry, see if you can understand what your baby wants you to know. Spend time being curious about who they are and what they are saying through their tiny movements, subtle (and not-so-subtle) sounds, and odd facial expressions. This small shift can give you a whole different experience of the postpartum period.

Your baby had a big experience, too. Everything is as new to them as it is to you right now. How can you support each other? Let your baby tell their story, and you tell yours. You need a safe space to tell your story and to process all the myriad changes you are feeling. Remember the hard work you did, and honor your body. Grieve for the things you might have wished were different. Give gratitude for what is your birth experience, for better or for worse. Search within until you can find the place of knowing, and trust that all is well and happened as it needed to. Give yourself and your baby the gifts of grace and time. Your birth was perfect. Exactly what your baby needed to begin their Earthside journey.

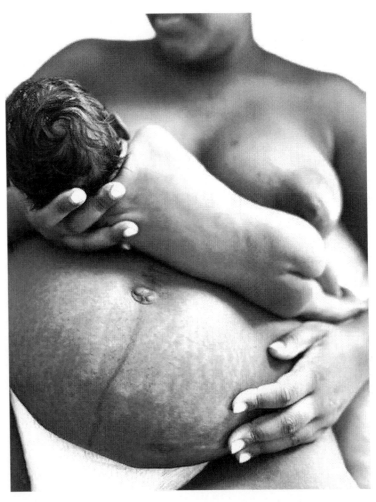

While your baby is inside, they have your undivided attention. You are with them 24/7. They're expecting that this will not change, once they are born. Your baby expects to still hear your heartbeat, smell and taste your breast milk, which smells and tastes similar to your amniotic fluid. They expect to be fed almost continuously, just like they were on the inside. Your breath regulates theirs. Your temperature regulates theirs.

Though they have heard the sounds of the outside world, the fast pace at which things move is completely foreign to them. Every single thing your baby sees, hears, touches, and smells is a new experience that they're integrating, as the millions of tiny neural pathways in their brain start to connect.

The first six weeks are the basis of the security your baby will feel for the rest of their lives. How does your baby want to spend these weeks? After everything has settled down from the birth, and you are tucked in your bed and have had the space to really breathe a sigh of relief for all of you have experienced during your birthing journey, take some moments just to be. Connect with your baby. Take some deep breaths. See baby's chest rise and fall, learn their rhythms. Spend several minutes just watching. When you feel you are on the same pacing as your baby, slow and easy, find that deep connection, your heart to your baby's heart. Ask what they need in this first six weeks. Where do they want to be, who do they want to see, what do they need to experience during this time?

The key to bonding with baby and healing after your birth is to s-l-o-w d-o-w-n. This was true prenatally, and it is even more true postnatally. Babies are on a completely different timeline than we are. They are still living outside of time as we know it. They do not have any sense of whether it is day or night or if something takes hours or minutes.

Let go of your own sense of time so you can fully appreciate your miraculous baby. Watch how slowly your baby does things. Seriously, turn off your phone and your TV, tune out the noise of your adult life, and watch your baby. They are fascinating. Every tiny, slow movement they make seems like a miracle—and it is! It is absolutely a miracle of God that two cells came together and, by some unknown force, grew into a fully functioning, unique human.

You have the rest of your life to be busy, to live by a clock, and to cram as much as you want into your hours. Right now, your only priority should be learning how to love and understand the baby that came out of your body. Let this be all that matters to you for forty days. It will change your life, heal your body and your heart, and ultimately make the world a safer place for all beings.

***

WOMB CONNECTION
PELVIC-FLOOR BREATHING

The way your body naturally works is that as you inhale, your lungs fill up with air, your diaphragm moves down, and all your internal organs shift slightly downward as your pelvic floor relaxes to give them room. As you exhale, your lungs deflate, everything shifts back upward, and your pelvic floor contracts.

Spend at least ten minutes every morning and ten minutes every night connecting with your pelvic floor. You may not be able to contract and relax with every breath when you first start, but you will be able to work up to that.

Sometimes, you may want to hold your baby as you do this and remember what it felt like for them and for you when they were in your womb, as you contract and relax these muscles that held them close inside. Other times, you may want to place one hand on your heart and one hand on your womb space, giving gratitude to your body for all the work it's done as you feel the healing taking place with each breath.

www.Genevamontano.com/WisdomFromTheWomb

***

THE MAGIC OF A BABY-LED BIRTH

I SAW EMEM TODAY. She and her son had finally come home from children's hospital two days ago.

This tiny heart warrior has battled a staph infection and RSV that he contracted because of his hospital stay. Once he was healthy enough to do catheter exploration, it was discovered that he has pulmonary atresia, and he was immediately operated on.

I cannot imagine the strength it takes as a mother to watch your brand-new baby battle these things, but I'm humbled by Emem's strength. She has never lost trust in her baby, not one time. She believes wholeheartedly that he knew he needed to wait longer before they operated, so he could grow stronger and bigger, and that is why he got sick two times.

She said, in her heart, she knew she would be in the hospital forty-five days. She just never wanted to say that number out loud, because it felt so long. She came home forty-five days after they went in. Her trust in God and in her baby have only grown stronger through this experience, and she makes me believe in the things I try to teach. She trusts and allows herself to be led by her baby in a way I can't honestly imagine in my own life, though I hope I would be as faithful. What a blessed baby.

I talked to Cammie, as well. Her wisdom is astounding. She sees truths about life and death that most of us will never understand. She sees how little control we have and graciously goes with the flow of motherhood. Honoring her struggles, while being grateful for the opportunity to be a mother.

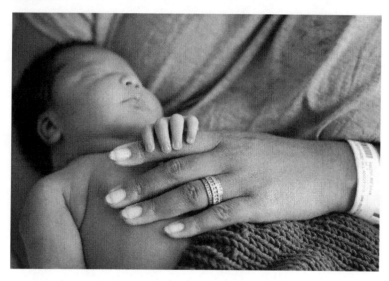

She misses her own mother and wishes they could all experience this time together. She wonders how long her son, a black male, will be cute, and when she will have to start worrying that he will be seen as a threat, have to start worrying for his safety every time he is outside her home. She says that remembering to shower saves her life some days. She is so clear in her gratitude to her baby for being here in her life, for choosing her. It is humbling.

Stephanie finished her six weeks of healing at home and feels really healthy and strong. Breastfeeding has been a challenge with this baby, and she is still taking her time, trying to learn what her baby needs and how this baby is different from her first.

As for me, my path continues, and though I often feel like I walk blindfolded, I trust I am held. In addition to midwifery, I am training new doulas and helping them learn how to support birthing people in a sacred way. We formed a non-profit with a mission to help end disparities among communities that experience harm during birth, while offering skills and training to people who can best support those communities. Knowing these new doulas can go out and create so much more good than I ever could by myself, brings me immense joy. We need doulas and midwives of color so that they can support their communities—the people who need support most in our culture. Proceeds from this book go to support this non-profit!

If you believe that babies and birthers should be heard, you owe it to them, to yourself, and to the world to get involved in birth or reproductive justice on a social or political level. Ask your insurance and state insurance to cover home birth, birth centers, all midwives, and doulas. Call your legislators. Believe in a person's right to choose when and how they become a parent. Support healers of all kinds. Don't give your money to people or organizations who don't listen to women or people of color. Speak up when you see injustices happening around you, at the hospital, at school, at the playground. Teach your babies about their bodies and about consent and how to use their voices. Find organizations that are already doing this work and give them your time or money. Become a doula. Do something. You are the person we have been waiting for. Let your baby inspire you to make a difference. If you aren't sure where to look, feel free to reach out to me personally.

I can't say I know where the path is leading next. I don't need to know. Just like in birth, I know I can never actually plan what the outcome will be. But I am excited. I am open. I am putting one foot in front of the other, and I know, wherever it leads, as long as I am listening to the quiet, I am where I am supposed to be.

As I am finishing this book, the world is uncertain around me. It is 2021. After the year 2020, which started out with clear vision, then *BOOM*! The coronavirus changed the way our world functions on a day-to-day basis. People are still uncertain whether they will have support people with them as they have their babies in a hospital. People are switching to home birth, because they are concerned for the safety of their babies. People are going to the hospital, facing the unknown, and learning the lessons they came to this life to learn. Decisions about vaccines divide families and communities.

It has been beautiful to realize that the preparation we do for birth and all the things I have written about in this book are valid for every uncertain situation in our lives. Birth is just like life! All the things I have reminded families during pregnancy and birth are the same things I reminded myself and my loved ones during the pandemic. Slow down. Take a breath. Whom or what do you trust?

Lean into those still, small voices that don't change. Ask yourself if there is something your soul wants to learn through this experience. Eat well, exercise, surround yourself with love, connect with your babies. We cannot control how your birth will go any more than we can control the spread of a virus or how it affects our economy, our well-being, and therefore our lives. But we can control our own choices. We can make the best of each moment and stay present with what is important.

I think about all I have learned over the years, from my clients, my teachers, and my children. I imagine what a world would be like if all babies knew that their parents really listen to them and trust them. Heck, I imagine what it would feel like if, as adults, we knew that our peers really listen and trust us! I honestly believe it would change the world, if true listening and connecting started from the time we were each in the womb. Or if parents had a true connection with their babies and trusted that their babies could communicate with them even before they had language. There would be so much less frustration amongst us, as a human race. We would feel so much more solid in our being, so much safer, knowing that from the moment we arrived into this body, we are heard.

I imagine how much easier parenting would be if we would truly listen to our babies. Sometimes, I have to laugh when I think about the things we do to babies because we don't understand them. I imagine, if I was having a rough day, maybe a stomach ache or maybe remembering something traumatic from the past, I imagine I might be tearful, and I would want to tell the people closest to me how I was feeling. I might not be my normal self. I might want to be alone, or I might want to be held.

What if, while I was trying to explain my feelings, the person I trust most in the world wrapped me up in a blanket super-tight, so I couldn't move, and shushed me every time I tried to speak. It makes me chuckle when I think about seeing my adult-size self swaddled and laid in my bed, so I can't move while my lover shushes me. But the truth is—I would be pissed. And I would be hurt down to the depths of my soul that I was so misunderstood. That, in my time of need, instead of being held and listened to, I was restrained and quieted, as if my voice didn't matter.

I don't know if this is how babies feel. But I do know that infants can communicate with us in ways we have forgotten. For example, your baby can communicate to you when they have had enough to eat. They are born with a built-in gas gauge. When they are hungry, their arms will be tense and flexed and their little fists will be close to their chests. As they fill up, their arms will relax, and once they are full, their arms and hands are loose and floppy and hang by their sides.

Babies have a different cry for when they are tired, hungry, upset, hurt, or bored. Parents who pay attention to their baby's cues can even learn to read when the baby needs to pee or poop and therefore don't have to use diapers. (It's called Elimination Communication—look it up!) Some parents have relearned how to listen to and be led by their babies on many different levels. They have learned how to make sleep routines easier, how the baby shows their various emotions, and the true capacity for communication that even the youngest babies possess. This is possible for all of us, if we take the time to slow down and listen to our babies.

And it is never too late! It is tempting to feel guilty, when we have older children, that we did not parent in a certain way when our kids were younger. Remember—your baby chose you as their parent. They wanted to experience exactly what you had to offer them at that moment in time. The lessons you were learning through them are not a coincidence or a mistake. If you want to do things differently now, you have that opportunity. It is never too late to slow down and listen.

I also know, as a parent, how frustrating it is when you're not sure why your baby is inconsolable. I, as a parent, have certainly had to put my baby down and walk away in order to maintain my sanity. But I wonder how it might have looked different if anyone had ever told me that my baby could communicate with me in a real way, if I could just slow down and listen. There are books written about how to communicate with toddlers and how to communicate with teenagers and how to calm a baby so they don't cry and how we, as adults, can learn to keep our cool.

I just can't help but wonder what it would be like if it started earlier. If we truly trust that these beings are infinite souls who have lived many lifetimes and are here to teach us something and to learn something themselves, how might we treat them differently?

If a stranger from another country, heck even another planet, came to your home and you did not understand their language or their ways, how would you treat them? I'm sure there would be times when there would be an incredible amount of frustration. But would we treat them the same way we do our babies? As if they know nothing and we are their superiors? Unfortunately, in this culture, I fear that we might. But maybe, if we had been respected as babies, that would look different today.

Some parents are afraid to trust their babies, because they feel like they are supposed to be the one who is strong and that, in trusting the baby to be the guide, they are neglecting their parental responsibilities to be the wise, authoritative teacher and role model. Some feel they would be draining their baby's positive energy from them, if they let baby lead.

Now that I have twenty years of parenting behind me with four different personalities, as well as having been a witness to many hundreds of parent-child relationships, I feel confident these parents will learn, as we all do, that the baby is here to teach us. We do best when we allow ourselves to lean into their peace, their courage, and their wisdom. We cannot drain these things from them, if we lean in with love and respect. They will merely help us rediscover our own peace, courage, and wisdom.

What we can teach our babies is to remain in the wisdom of their fetal self. To find slow, quiet moments. To make decisions based on a pause. To take the time they need to listen and understand the people around them, to understand themselves. We can teach them that all people deserve to be heard. That all people have something valuable to contribute. We can remind them they are here to change the world. They came specifically to fulfill a greater purpose, and we support them in finding that no matter what. We can teach them to be humble and to ask for forgiveness often. We can teach them they are enough, that they don't always have to get it right, and that the mistakes they make will make them great.

Your baby is magical. I hope from the depths of my heart you will take the time to experience this magic. It takes time and a relearning of what we think we know about pregnancy and birth. It takes a different level of responsibility to your birth than many people are willing to take. It takes a willingness to move more slowly than you have since you were inside your own mother's womb. It takes a commitment to your own healing.

Nine months, forty days, and a lifetime of you and your baby gazing into one another's spirits as you prepare to open your body, die and be reborn, then allow your birth wounds to close up as your baby prepares to start experiencing their own wounds, so they can begin learning the lessons they came for, heal their ancestors, and change the world.

I hope from the depths of my heart that you will create the opportunity to experience the true magic of being led by your baby's wisdom.

***

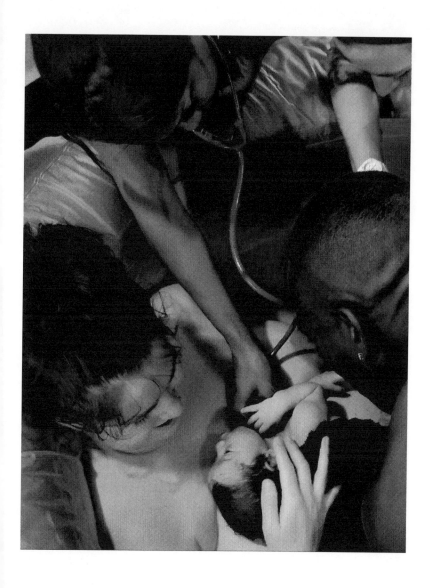

ACKNOWLEDGMENTS

AS A FEMALE-BODIED PERSON, I have the honor and privilege of creating life. I am, first and foremost, forever grateful to my children, Liv, Dre, Shiloh, and Eden. Thank you for choosing me as your mother, for the lessons you have taught me and continue to teach me. As you grow from seeds to saplings to towering oaks, it is a blessing to plant new seeds in my creative spaces.

My blossoming midwifery practice and doula training program are two such sprouts that I currently have the joy of cultivating. I always knew I would write a book, and planting its seeds and watching it gestate has been a gift.

I am forever grateful to my teachers and mentors, Sena Johnson, Melissa Sexton, Margie McSweeney, Penny Lyon, Nataline Cruz, Kristin Schuch, Somah McCracken, and to my ride-or-dies, Lucia Fellers, Amy Haderer, Natalie McAnulla, Whitney Nichols, and my parents, Lola Carter, Wayne Klahn, Pat Biel, and Vina Johnson. Each one of you has played such an important part in my story, and without the blessings you have bestowed on my life, I could never be where I am today. Your love has made a difference.

Lastly, I have to thank every baby who has given me the opportunity to help them out. The magic you bring to the garden of this world is what keeps it growing.

ABOUT THE AUTHOR

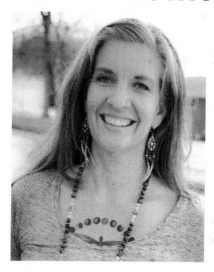

GENEVA MONTANO is a Colorado native and mother of four. She has been a birth worker since 2003 and has attended over 650 births in homes, birth centers, and hospitals. Geneva has had a lifelong passion for spirituality, art, and self-exploration. She believes that each birth teaches her and the families she serves the life lessons they have been seeking.

Geneva is a Registered and Certified Professional Midwife, Certified Doula,

Registered Yoga teacher, prenatal and postnatal yoga teacher, CPR instructor, body and energy worker, doula trainer, author, artist, and activist. She is certified in womb massage, holistic healing of the pregnant and postpartum bodies, NLP, quantum transformation, and more. She loves teaching, listening to people's stories with her ears, heart, and hands, and being a vessel for transmitting divine healing to bodies and spirits.

Midwife. Doula. Spirit Medicine.

www.GenevaMontano.com

RESOURCES MENTIONED

Authors:
Ina May Gaskin
Pam England
Gurmukh
Debra Pascali Bonnaro
Emily Oster
Henci Goer
Kimberly Ann Johnson
Heng Ou

Videos:
Orgasmic Birth
Jim Gaffigan—Mr. Universe
Why Not Home
Business of Being Born

Websites/Apps:
FreeBirthSociety.com
IndieBirth.org
Spinningbabies.com
MotherboardBirth.com
EvidenceBasedBirth.com

Services:
Institute for Birth Healing
Mayan abdominal massage
Webster certified chiropractic care
Hypnosis for Birth

Birth photography credits:
Aperture Grrl Photography
Rebecca Ann Walsh Photography/Birth Becomes Her
Taylor Davenport Photography
Forest Joy, Moon Child Doula

ENDNOTES

[1] Michaela D. Filiou, Max Planck Institute of Psychiatry, Germany; Maria Syrrou, Laboratory of Biology, Faculty of Medicine, School of Health Sciences, University of Ioannina, Greece. *Stressful Newborn Memories: Pre-Conceptual, In Utero, and Postnatal Events* www.frontiersin.org/article/10.3389/fpsyt.2019.00220.

[2] Petersen EE, Davis NL, Goodman D, et al. "Racial/Ethnic Disparities in Pregnancy-Related Deaths - United States, 2007–2016." *MMWR Morb Mortal Weekly Report* 2019;68:762–765. DOI: http://dx.doi.org/10.15585/mmwr.mm6835a3.

[3] Grobman WA, Rice MM, Reddy UM, Tita ATN, Silver RM, Mallett G, Hill K, Thom EA, El-Sayed YY, Perez-Delboy A, Rouse DJ, Saade GR, Boggess KA, Chauhan SP, Iams JD, Chien EK, Casey BM, Gibbs RS, Srinivas SK, Swamy GK, Simhan HN, Macones GA; Eunice Kennedy Shriver National Institute of Child Health and Human Development Maternal-Fetal Medicine Units Network. "Labor Induction versus Expectant Management in Low-Risk Nulliparous Women." *New England Journal of Medicine*. 2018 Aug 9;379(6):513-523. doi: 10.1056/NEJMoa1800566.

[4] Ross S, Bossis A, Guss J, Agin-Liebes G, Malone T, Cohen B, Mennenga SE, Belser A, Kalliontzi K, Babb J, Su Z, Corby P, Schmidt BL. "Rapid and sustained symptom reduction following psilocybin treatment for anxiety and depression in patients with life-threatening cancer: a randomized controlled trial." *Journal of Psychopharmacology*. 2016 Dec;30(12):1165-1180. doi: 10.1177/0269881116675512. PMID: 27909164; PMCID: PMC5367551.

5 Makary M A, Daniel M. "Medical error—the third leading cause of death in the US." *BMJ* 2016; 353i2139 doi:10.1136/bmj.i2139.

6 Jane Sandall et al., "Midwife-Led Continuity Models Versus Other Models of Care for Childbearing Women," *Cochrane Database System Review.* 4 (Apr. 28, 2016): CD004667.

7 Cheyney, M., Bovbjerg, M., Everson, M. A., et al. (2014). "Outcomes of care for 16,924 planned home births in the United States: The Midwives Alliance of North America Statistics Project, 2004 to 2009." *Journal of Midwifery Women's Health* 59(1): 17-27.

8 Miranda, MD, Navio, C. "Benefits of Exercise for Pregnant Women." *Journal of Sport and Health Research* 2013 Vol.5 No.2 pp.229-232 ref.4.

9 Sutton, Jean and Scott, Pauline. "Understanding and Teaching Optimal Foetal Positioning." *New Zealand: Birth Concepts*, 1995.

10 Declercq ER, Sakala C, Corry MP, Applebaum S. "Listening to Mothers II: Report of the Second National U.S. Survey of Women's Childbearing Experiences: Conducted January-February 2006 for Childbirth Connection by Harris Interactive(R) in partnership with Lamaze International." *Journal of Perinatal Education.* 2007 Fall;16(4):15-7. doi: 10.1624/105812407X244778. PMID: 18769522; PMCID: PMC2174391.

11 Amis D. "Healthy birth practice #1: let labor begin on its own." *Journal of Perinatal Education.* 2014;23(4):178-187. doi:10.1891/1058-1243.23.4.178.

12 Young SM, Gryder LK, Zava D, Kimball DW, Benyshek DC. "Presence and concentration of 17 hormones in human placenta processed for encapsulation and consumption." *Placenta.* 2016 Jul;43:86-9. doi: 10.1016/j.placenta.2016.05.005.

Young SM, Gryder LK, David WB, Teng Y, Gerstenberger S, Benyshek DC. "Human placenta processed for encapsulation contains modest concentrations of 14 trace minerals and elements." *Nutrition Research.* 2016 Aug;36(8):872-8. doi: 10.1016/j.nutres.2016.04.005.

13 van Rheenen P. "Delayed cord clamping and improved infant outcomes." *BMJ* 2011; 343 :d7127 doi:10.1136/bmj.d7127.

14 "Guideline: counselling of women to improve breastfeeding practices." Geneva: World Health Organization; 2018. License: CC BY-NC-SA 3.0 IGO.

15 Elizabeth Werner, Maia Miller, Lauren M. Osborne, Sierra Kuzava, Catherine MonkArch. *Women's Mental Health.* Author manuscript; available in PMC 2016 Feb 1. Published in final edited form as:

Arch Women's Mental Health. 2015 Feb; 18(1): 41–60. Published online 2014 Nov 25. doi: 10.1007/s00737-014-0475-y PMCID: PMC4308451.